HOW TO
DIE IN THE
OUTDOORS

HOW TO DIE IN THE OUTDOORS

150 WILD WAYS to PERISH

THIRD EDITION

BUCK TILTON, MS, MA

ILLUSTRATIONS BY ROBERT L. PRINCE

FALCON®

GUILFORD, CONNECTICUT

For the ones who truly make me want to go on living,
my family: Kat, Amber, McKenzie, Zachary, and Bo

FALCON®

An imprint of Globe Pequot
Falcon, FalconGuides, and Make Adventure Your Story are registered trademarks of
Rowman & Littlefield.

Distributed by NATIONAL BOOK NETWORK

Illustrations: Robert Prince | www.robertlprince.com

British Library Cataloguing in Publication Information Available

Library of Congress Cataloging-in-Publication Data
Tilton, Buck.
  How to die in the outdoors : from bad bears to toxic toads, 150 grizzly ways to croak /
Buck Tilton. — 3rd ed.
    p. cm.
  ISBN 978-0-7627-5410-6
  1. Outdoor medical emergencies—Prevention. I. Title.
  RC88.9.O95T54 2010
  616.02'52—dc22
2009022540
ISBN 978-1-4930-2783-5 (paperback)
ISBN 978-1-4930-2784-2 (e-book)

∞™ The paper used in this publication meets the minimum requirements of American
National Standard for Information Sciences—Permanence of Paper for Printed Library
Materials, ANSI/NISO Z39.48-1992.

CONTENTS

DEATH BY MERCILESS MAMMAL

DEATH BY BODACIOUS BIRD

DEATH BY AQUATIC ACCIDENT

DEATH BY POISONOUS PLANT

DEATH BY DISASTROUS DISEASE

DEATH BY NEFARIOUS NATURE

DEATH BY SPITEFUL SPIDER

DEATH BY FICKLE FATE

INTRODUCTION

Man dies when he wants,
as he wants, of what he chooses.

JEAN ANOUILH, 1960

Anyone can die of heart disease. In the United States, in fact, most people do. The process is time consuming but simple. All you have to do is eat a lot of fat, give up exercise, smoke cigarettes, drink heavily (not water), worry, and watch the quality of your life fade into oblivion. After a while you'll experience chest pain and shortness of breath, the old ticker will tick its last, and you'll collapse on the living room floor, on the bathroom floor, or into your mashed potatoes. How very uninteresting!

During the last year for which accurate records are available, there were, rounded off, 2.6 million human deaths registered in the 50 sort of United States. These are the Big 10 ways "We the People," and people in other highly developed countries, expired over the past 10 years:

Heart disease
Stroke
Chronic obstructive pulmonary disease
Lower respiratory diseases
Tracheal, bronchus, and lung cancers
HIV/AIDS
Diarrheal diseases
Diabetes

Motor vehicle accidents

Hypertensive diseases

Basically, if you live a normal, boring life like most everybody does, staying indoors most of the time, spending your leisure hours involved in activities that do little or nothing to promote health, you have an excellent chance of ending up somewhere on this list. Meanwhile in the outdoors, close to the natural world, of which you are far more a part than you may realize, there are numerous interesting ways to perish: by snake bite, crab claw, elephant foot, walrus tusk, rhino horn, and many, many more.

What you'll read about in this book concerns not only the details of how you can die—some of the ways intriguingly painful and/or gory, and all based (more or less) on facts—but also ways to avoid death should life-threatening situations arise in which you decide you are not ready to check out of this world and into whatever afterlife there may be.

The author has taken great pains, figuratively speaking, to keep you interested. So, read on, enjoy . . . and live!

DEATH BY
RAPACIOUS
REPTILE

Within the class Reptilia, scientists list about 10,000 species, including the snakes, lizards, crocodilians, and turtles. Frogs and toads are of the class Amphibia but are herein lumped with reptiles because . . . well, they just are. Just so you know, some scientists think birds and reptiles belong in the same class. Watch for it. Over the millennia reptiles have developed the same basic defensive stance. Not really a "stance," what they do is run and hide. If pressured, however, and in some cases if they are hungry enough, a few reptiles will attack and kill a human being. This section is about pressured and hungry reptiles.

ATTACKED BY ALLIGATOR

Death cancels everything but truth.

ANONYMOUS

Back when life on earth was young, millions of years ago, alligators crawled or swam over the entire landmass we call the United States. These creatures and their relatives (see "Crunched by Crocodile") have changed little, but the weather changed, people got pushy, and now the American alligator (*Alligator mississippiensis*) is relegated to a relatively small area: coastal Virginia south to Florida, west to Texas, and up the Mississippi River to southern Arkansas. They prefer life wet and mucky in marshes and swamps, in muddy rivers and lakes, and sometimes at the edge of the ocean. They also like it hot, but unlike other crocodilians, alligators will survive temperatures down to the 30s Fahrenheit, although they go dormant in the cold. Mature alligators, when conditions are just right, have reached almost 20 feet in length and over 1,000 pounds in weight.

American alligators can live contentedly for long periods of time between meals. When they are ready to eat, they go out exclusively for a meat dinner, choosing, whenever possible, something bite-size that they can swallow whole, large fish and birds being at the top of the menu. Being unable to chew, alligators must tear anything too big to swallow into swallow-able chunks, an energy-consuming endeavor these reptiles would rather avoid. Alligators, therefore, rarely take a bite out of humans, and if they do, they are always very upset or very hungry. In the last 60 years or so, alligators have killed about two dozen humans in the United States—roughly one person every two and a half years. Small adults and children are at a much higher risk for becoming alligator food.

Why You Die

Alligators are experts at attacking. Swimming below the surface of the water, only their eyeballs exposed, they silently approach their prey, gambling everything on one swift and merciless strike. If the attackee happens to be you, your first awareness of danger will most likely be the snapping of powerful jaws as they close over a bite-able body part, arm or leg, and the unusual feel of long teeth sinking deep into your flesh. Alligators then rotate rapidly along the length of their axis until the part of you they are tenaciously holding rips off. You may not feel pain yet, but you will feel the gush of your blood from the hole where a part of you was recently attached. If your arm or leg was small, the alligator will be back for more. Then the uneaten part of you will be dragged below the surface and stuffed under a log or into a hole in a muddy bank so the alligator can rip off more pieces as the need to eat dictates. Fortunately, you will drown long before you succumb to the pain and horror.

To Live

Give alligators plenty of personal space: Fatal encounters occur most often when someone intentionally messes with one. Alligators have attacked humans who got too close to nests and eggs, and adult alligators will attack to defend baby gators, sometimes even when the babies are not their own. Stay dry: As a close second to people who mess with them, alligators attack people swimming with them. If bitten, strike vigorously at the nose, and the alligator may release you. If you are bitten and survive, find a doctor soon. Alligators have dirty mouths.

> Moral: Always swim with someone substantially smaller than you.

2 ATTENUATED BY ANACONDA

> Is life a boon? If so, it must befall that Death,
> whene'er he call, must call too soon.
>
> W. S. GILBERT, 1888

Of the six species of giant snakes now living on earth, none grows larger than the green anaconda (*Eunectes murinus*), which might surpass 40 feet in length. Living only in the rivers and swamps of South America, the anaconda swims with great agility and speed, a formidable and slim torpedo that can weigh over 400 pounds. Anacondas cannot see well, but they "hear" through their skull bones and "smell" with flicks of their tongues. Their jaws can separate a long way north-south and east-west, ending up attached to the snake only by elastic ligaments.

Why You Die

An anaconda will bite you first with a large mouth full of sharp teeth that curve backwards, allowing the snake to hang on, sometimes despite your most vigorous attempts to dislodge it. Terrible but not toxic, the bite becomes the least of your worries as the snake coils its body around yours. Despite myths to the contrary, it is unlikely any of your bones will be broken, a fact that will give you very little comfort. Each time you exhale, and exhale you must, the snake tightens its grip until you are no longer able to draw breath. No breath, no life.

If you are unusually small, the anaconda will then unhinge its mouth to a prodigious width and swallow you whole. The digestion process will take a week or more depending on your size. If you happen to be too big to swallow, lucky you, you will be left dead and useless to the snake. What a waste!

To Live

Anaconda attacks on humans are rare, and even more rarely fatal—although a few encounters are believed to have been predatory in nature. The snake, in other words, was seeking food. If attacked, you will most likely be able to fight free, though bloodied and bruised, especially if someone is there to help you.

Moral: Never hug anything that eats human flesh.

3 | BITTEN BY BEADED LIZARD

Men fear death, as children fear
to go in the dark . . .

FRANCIS BACON, 1625

They are tagged as "beaded" due to their bumpy skin, each bump or "bead" containing a tiny bit of bone. Collectively, these bumps give the lizards something arguably akin to armor. Their scientific name, *Heloderma horridum*, tells you they have studded skin (*Heloderma*) and they are horrible (*horridum*). "Horrible," of course, remains somewhat subjective—your horrible might not be so to someone else. The female may reach 30 inches and tip a scale to 5 pounds. The male could be 6 inches longer and a pound or so heavier. Extraordinary males have reached nearly 10 pounds. Often called Mexican beaded lizards, they range over a large part of central and western Mexico, as the name might at least suggest, and down into Guatemala, and they are almost always found in forests: tropical, scrub, and pine. One of only two venomous lizards on earth, the beaded lizard is shaped similarly to a Gila monster (the other venomous lizard), but grows larger and displays less color on its skin than a Gila monster, with the beaded lizard commonly dark. Beaded lizards and Gila monsters have venoms that are pretty much the same.

Why You Die

A bite will cause pain, quite a heap of it. You can turn red and swell up where the lizard bit you, and you may start sweating. It's more serious if your heart rate increases more than a little, you begin to hemorrhage internally, and your blood pressure decreases. The really serious bad thing will be respiratory failure.

To Live

Your death will be the result of your forgetting the cardinal rule of encounters with venomous creatures, which is leave them alone—so leave them alone. As with Gila monsters, beaded lizards don't like to let go after they bite. You need to make them let go (see "Held Up by Gila Monster"). Then clean the wound and find a doctor.

Moral: Leave the beadwork to those
skilled with needle and thread.

4   BAFFLED BY BOUGA TOAD

Death takes away the commonplace of life.
ALEXANDER SMITH, 1863

Amphibians (toads, frogs, salamanders) are descended from the first creatures to squirm out of the water and take up residence on land, something that began to happen more than 280 million years ago, and they still occupy that mysterious interzone position: half land animal, half water animal. Of all the groups of vertebrates, amphibians are the most benign to humans. They destroy nothing we want, transmit no known diseases, eat tons of obnoxious insects, and have no venomous bites. A few species, however, can cause death to humans in unusual ways.

The skin of nearly all amphibians secretes some poison, a device they apparently use to protect themselves from something that might eat them (see "Finalized by Frog"). Some species—notably the bouga toad (genus *Bufo*), a Caribbean resident colored in all the tints of leaf litter, chubby and warty in typical toad fashion—secrete a hallucinogen used by the ancient Mayans, modern Central Americans, and Haitian shamans. The toads are against such uses. They get thrown in a pot of boiling water, which forces the juice out of glands behind their eyes. After boiling, the toads are removed dead from the pot. The person who drinks the brew drops over as if dead but resurrects soon to wander around zombielike, doing the bidding of a medicine man or witch doctor until the toad tea wears off.

Why You Die

A toad too many, or a swallow too many, and the person who drinks the brew enters a coma from which there is no resurrection. More unappealing, people under the influence of bouga juice have seemed so dead they were buried . . . still alive.

To Live

Do not touch bouga toads with your hands or your mouth.

Moral: Too many toads spoil the broth.

5   BURIED BY BROWN SNAKE

> To die is different from what any
> one supposed, and luckier.
>
> WALT WHITMAN, 1855

Attaching the name "brown" to a snake does little to describe anything in particular. The smallish North American brown snake, for instance, can be yellowish and sometimes spotted and, more important in this context, packs no poison.

Here our interest lies with the Australian brown snake, one of the most venomous in the world. But misunderstanding may still arise since there are at present nine species, and a few subspecies, of genus *Pseudonaja* crawling about Australia and New Guinea. They all, however, are long (growing often to 6 feet and as much as 8 feet) with narrow heads. They are also typically and uniformly brown in color— although you may see patterns of color variations from basic brown, especially in juvenile snakes (that are also capable of fatally biting a grown-up human). Since they do not mind, or at least do tolerate, living near people, and since they are easily upset, brown snakes are responsible for the most poisonous snakebites in Australia. Brown snake fangs are not very long, which is good, and they tend to inject a relatively small amount of venom, which is also good. And sometimes the bites are "dry" or lacking a deposit of venom, and that's even better.

Why You Die

Things are not good when you get a big blast of the neurotoxic venom, which most often comes from a big brown snake. Australia's eastern brown, a large species, has been called, by some experts, the second most deadly land snake on earth. Your sudden collapse not long after a bite would not be uncommon. If you stay conscious, you may have a lot of pain, some of it in your abdomen, along with dizziness, difficulty breathing and swallowing, and a drop in blood pressure. You may bleed uncontrollably, and you may die because your heart has stopped working.

To Live

Keep still and apply the pressure-immobilization bandage described in "Terrified by Taipan." Once on, do not take the bandage off. And send for a doctor.

Moral: If it's brown, leave it down.

COLLAPSED BY CAIMAN

> How little room do we take up in death,
> that, living, know no bounds.
>
> JAMES SHIRLEY, 1626

An alligatorid of Central and South America, caimans swim in slow, freshwater rivers and lakes, and in marshy areas, and they vary in size from the dwarf caiman (*Paleosuchus palpebrosus*), which usually quits growing at 3 feet or so in length, up through more than a half dozen species to the black caiman (*Melanosuchus niger*), which could reach 20 feet. At 20 feet—and even when it is a few feet less—the scaly black caiman ranks as the largest predator of the Amazon basin. Large caimans, in fact, never worry about being prey themselves unless they are stalked by humans. In some areas these reptiles have been hunted, for their skin and meat, to near extinction. Caimans all look a lot like alligators, but caimans have boney plates buried in the skin of their underside and longer, skinnier, and possibly more pointed teeth than alligators. Those teeth are designed for grabbing and holding, which is what they do to their prey, almost always underwater until the animal-to-be-eaten drowns. Preferring a diet of fresh fish with an occasional bird or mammal (such as a capybara or a monkey), caimans, like alligators, cannot chew—so they have to swallow their food whole.

Why You Die

If you are in water, the caiman will pull you under and hold on until you are dead. If you are on land, the caiman will exert a great deal of energy in order to drag you into water. In both events, should the caiman be successful, you will be torn apart and devoured.

To Live

Stay out of water known to be frequented by caimans. If you end up in water with one, swim to land as quickly and quietly as possible. Noise, such as screaming, and thrashing interest them. If you see one on land, run away. If one gets hold of you, in water or on land, go for the eyes, its most sensitive spot. If that is not working, reach into the reptile's mouth and try to grab the palatal valve, a flap of skin at the back of the tongue that prevents water from entering the animal's airway. Yank on the flap, and you should be released. And good luck with that last suggestion.

> Moral: Never feed wild animals,
> especially with parts of yourself.

7 | CROAKED BY CANE TOAD

He hath lived ill that knows not how to die well.

THOMAS FULLER, 1732

At 4 to 9 inches long and up to 4 pounds in weight, cane toads (*Bufo marinus*) are big and fat, greenish yellow, and able to put rabbits to shame with their ability to reproduce. A pair of cane toads would produce 60,000 more toadies every year if all their eggs became mature adults. These amphibians were imported once upon a time from South America to Australia to eat beetles attacking sugarcane fields. Hopping rampant and feeding at night, they took a liking to Down Under and proliferated to the point where they're thicker than fleas on a dingo's back. In addition to insects, cane toads will eat meat, including small birds and each other. Crushed, the toads stink vilely, but that's only a small part of the problem.

Why You Die

Two glands on the sides of their wart-strewn bodies constantly secrete venom called bufotenine. When the toads are pressured, the secretion rate increases, and when they are really upset, the venom shoots out up to 40 inches, causing temporary blindness if it lands in your eye. Anything attempting to eat a cane toad, a really upsetting experience for the toad, dies from the venom. A growing number of humans with questionable intelligence remove and dry the toad's skin and smoke it for what is reportedly an acceptable high. A growing number of the growing number are dying: The venom causes respiratory difficulties and slows one's heart rate enough to cause death. On the ragged edge of humanity, a few have actually licked the toad for the hallucinogenic effect. Now there's an interesting way to croak.

To Live

Obviously, avoid any contact with cane toads. But if you fail to follow this advice, get to a hospital. A dose of digoxin to speed up your heart might work.

Moral: Toads can take a licking
and keep on kicking.

8   CLOBBERED BY COBRA

> Death will not see me flinch; the heart is
> bold that pain has made incapable of pain.
>
> DOROTHY PARKER, 1926

The Elapidae family of snakes includes about 230 species, many of them cobras, and all elapids are venomous. Few snakes on earth, maybe none, have received as much publicity as cobras, inhabitants of Africa and Asia, distinctive partially due to their impressive "hoods," which fan out from their necks via special little rib bones. The famous asp of Egypt, killer of Cleopatra, immortalized in so many statues, is an Egyptian cobra (*Naja haje*). The fascinating snake charmers of India musically charm common cobras (*Naja naja*), which rise up sinuously from baskets. The mighty king cobra (*Ophiophagus hannah*), measured at almost 19 feet in length, is the world's largest venomous snake and possesses an extremely deadly bite at least partly due to its great size.

Cobras all possess short, hollow, fixed fangs and neurotoxic venom (which means the venom attacks the central nervous system instead of rushing around in the blood and causing damage the way a hemotoxic venom does). Cobras, the king cobra being an exception, generally don't mind living near and biting humans on a regular basis.

Another universally feared elapid is the black-neck spitting cobra (*Naja nicricollis*), an irascible animal with the nasty habit of literally spitting its venom from holes in the front of its fangs distances up to about 7 feet with great accuracy. It always aims for the eyes, and the venom causes severe pain and blindness long enough for the snake to slither in for a deadly bite.

Why You Die

You'll feel pain when a cobra bites, and you'll swell near the bite, get weak and drowsy, have trouble seeing and swallowing, develop a headache, and lose your ability to talk. Then you'll drool, throw up, become numb and partially paralyzed, and convulse before you slip into complete paralysis, including that of the muscles that power your breathing—so you die.

To Live

Retreat as soon as possible to a medical facility where advanced care, including airway support and antivenin, is available. If a spitting cobra's venom hits your eye, wash it out with copious amounts of water.

Moral: If it slithers, run away.

CORRALLED BY CORAL SNAKE

> The nearest friends can go with anyone
> to death, comes so far short they
> might as well not try to go at all.
>
> ROBERT FROST, 1914

All of the poisonous snakes in the United States are members of either the family Crotalidae (see "Reaped by Rattlesnake") or the family Elapidae, which includes, in North America, two genera: *Micrurus* (the southeastern, Florida, and Texas coral snakes) and *Micruroides* (the Sonoran coral snake). Among the most brightly colorful animals on the continent, coral snakes are banded in brilliant red, yellow, and shiny black. They are often confused with the equally colorful and harmless scarlet king snake, but the order of the colors differs. If red is bordered on both sides by black, the snake will not harm you. If red is bordered on both sides by yellow (or sometimes white), the snake is venomous.

Slim and rarely reaching 2 feet in length, without an enlarged head, coral snakes are shy and reclusive, with a primitive venom system that includes two short, fixed, relatively dull fangs in the front of the upper jaw. They cannot strike out and rip through clothing and, indeed, must literally chew for several seconds in order to break your skin and shoot you up with very potent neurotoxic venom.

Why You Die

Human deaths are rare since most people yank off the snake before it gnaws through their skin. If you are silly enough to let a coral snake gnaw its way through your skin, you probably will feel little or no pain and see no swelling. From 90 minutes to as much as 12 hours later, however, you should start to feel weak or numb, especially in the bitten arm or leg. A few hours later you will start to drool and shake. You may feel drowsy. At some point you'll find it difficult to talk and then breathe. When you can't breathe at all, you'll die.

To Live

In case of a bite, wrap your whole arm or leg in an elastic bandage, firmly but not tight enough to cut off circulation. Splint the arm or leg and get carried to a doctor ASAP.

> **Moral:** Red on yellow kills a
> fellow . . . or a woman.

10 CRUNCHED BY CROCODILE

It is as natural to die as to be born.

FRANCIS BACON, 1625

True remnants of the Age of Reptiles, the only living descendants of the most successful class of land vertebrates ever, crocodiles and their relatives (see "Attacked by Alligator") have changed little in the last 70 million years or so. One alteration in crocodiles is that they once grew to more than 50 feet in length. Today, if you're lucky . . . or unlucky . . . you may see a crocodile (*Crocodylus acutus, Crocodylus intermedius*) reaching 23 feet from snout to end of powerful tail. They like their weather really hot and are found in all tropical regions on earth: northern South America, southern North America, Africa, India, Southeast Asia, northern Australia, and other such places.

No animals, with the possible exception of a few sharks (see "Gobbled by Great White Shark") and polar bears (see "Pulverized by Polar Bear"), are as totally dedicated to eating meat. On a lazy day, when the pickings are slim, crocodiles are well-known devourers of their own young.

The smell of blood immediately arouses crocodiles. They will slide silently and efficiently into the water, approaching a bleeding victim with immense strokes of their tails even when they aren't especially hungry. Far more aggressive and voracious than their alligator cousins, crocodiles think

nothing of attacking something quite a bit bigger than themselves. In regions of the world where registration of the dead
is not required, crocodiles crunch humans regularly, even
pulling them from small boats on the Nile River and spurting
up to 50 yards onto land to pull down slow runners.

Why You Die

Like alligators, crocs can't chew. Having taken hold, they, like
alligators, will rotate rapidly along the length of their axis
until the part of you they are gripping rips off to be swallowed
whole. They will almost always still be hungry and back for
more. In fact, they are fond of tucking food away underwater

for a snack later. If you happen to be tough, your storage for later consumption softens you up for added delectability and easier dismemberment.

To Live

Crocodiles have occasionally been driven off by repeated and aggressive thumps to their snout.

> Moral: The only safe crocodile
> lives somewhere you aren't.

11 ERADICATED BY EUROPEAN VIPER

> One thing is sure; there are just two
> respectable ways to die. One is of old
> age, and the other is by accident.
>
> ELBERT HUBBARD, PROBABLY 1895

Among several claims to fame, this snake is the only venomous one in Great Britain. Its range, however, extends all across Europe and well into Asia, reaching both Mongolia and parts of China. Typically about 2 feet in length, it can measure up to almost 3 feet, and it is thick of body with sides that slope off nearly vertically. Its head is distinctly wider than where that head joins the body. It can be almost entirely black or brown or lighter in color with interesting and intricate patterns, such as a zigzaggy line of a darker color on its back. This snake can hunker down comfortably in a great a variety of habitats, from French coastal dunes to Swiss Alps to Russian steppes. Depending on where you are, local people might refer to it by numerous names, including common viper and common adder as well as European viper, but *Vipera berus* (yay for Latin) applies to all these serpents.

Often described as timid, these snakes avoid encounters with humans whenever possible. Those bitten usually step on the viper, accidentally, or pick one up, nonaccidentally. Even then, generally speaking, this viper rates low on the you-might-die scale. The venom is not super powerful. In

Britain there is a viper-related fatality about once per decade. In some other countries the death rate is even lower.

Why You Die

The immediate and intense pain, though undesirable, will not harm you. Swelling comes next, followed by tingling. The pain and swelling may extend from the bite site for several hours, and then subside after, oh, 24 hours. The unusual severe shock and occasional cardiac arrest are more likely in small children.

To Live

Even though your chances of living are very good, a visit to a medical facility is certainly a wise use of your time. At least eight types of antivenin are available, and they are all pretty much effective.

> **Moral:** An accident can be premeditated carelessness.

FINALIZED BY FROG

Even the bold will fly when they see Death
drawing in close enough to end their life.

SOPHOCLES, ABOUT 442 BCE

Quite a few members of the South and Central American frog families of Atelopidae and Dendrobatidae are the most poisonous of the world's amphibians, especially the latter, the arrow-poison frogs (sometimes called poison-dart frogs). Most frogs and toads have skin with some degree of poison in it (see "Baffled by Bouga Toad"), but nothing as potent as arrow-poison frogs, whose skin may actually contain one of the most potent biotoxins in the animal kingdom.

Brightly colorful and reportedly dangerous to handle even casually, these amphibians are also small, some reaching maturity at less than an inch in length. They are carefully gathered by South American Indians who are fond of roasting poison-arrow frogs on sticks over an open fire. The poison that drips off the sizzling amphibian is collected and concocted into a potion that the Indians use to coat their arrow tips and blow darts to increase their chances of a kill while hunting. Some species of arrow-poison frogs have skin so poisonous the Indians simply pin the creature to the forest floor and rub the points of their weapons along the backs of the frogs. Thus the name—and thus another reason to stay on friendly terms with as many fellow earthlings as possible.

Why You Die

Not much is known about the vitality of frog poison since human volunteers for scientific experiments related to why and how fast you die are hard to come by. What seems to happen is this: You get frog poison inside you, and your heart speeds up until it's going so fast that blood cannot refill the chambers between beats—so it stops. Convulsions may add a touch of interest to your final moments.

To Live

Unfortunately, there is no known antidote—so don't touch any colorful little frogs or South American arrowheads.

Moral: Look, but don't touch.

HELD UP BY GILA MONSTER

> To die completely, a person must not
> only forget but be forgotten, and he
> who is not forgotten is not dead.
>
> SAMUEL BUTLER, ABOUT 1902

About 3,000 species of lizards are known today, most of them harmless to humans. Only two species are venomous—despite plenty of mythology to the contrary—and therefore potentially lethal via poison. The deadly ones are the beaded lizard (see "Bitten by Beaded Lizard") and the Gila monster, both of genus *Heloderma*, the Gila monster being specifically *Heloderma suspectum*.

While the venom glands of snakes are in their upper jaws, the venom glands of these lizards are in their lower jaws and not connected to the teeth (as in snakes). These lizards must grab hold and chew the venom into the wound they make. Due to the lack of a venom injection system, these lizards use stubborn stick-to-itiveness.

Gila (hee-lah) monsters live quiet and peaceful lives, hunting at night throughout northern Mexico and the southwestern United States, and they grow to almost 2 feet in length. They are essentially black with broad smears of yellow and pink. Because they carry a neurotoxin in their venom, Gila monsters would not normally cause much pain when they bite but for the fact that they hang on so tightly and chew so hard. They never bite humans unless they are messed with, at which time they are capable of pivoting rapidly on their hind legs and lashing out with incredible speed.

Why You Die

If they work enough venom into the wound, you'll see some swelling. You may feel numb and weak. You'll feel your heart speed up. You'll probably vomit, feel dizzy, and have increasing difficulty breathing. Bitten humans most often survive, but if you don't it will be because you are not breathing enough to stay alive.

To Live

Once bitten, remove the Gila monster as soon as possible. This may require cutting the jaw muscles of the lizard. Applications of high heat, such as from a cigarette lighter, to the underside of the jaw have also worked. Then, just to be safe, find a doctor.

Moral: Not all monsters are in the movies.

14 | KREAMED BY KOMODO DRAGON

Death always comes too early or too late.

ENGLISH PROVERB

Lying about 240 miles east of Bali in Indonesia, Komodo is a desolate, volcanic, "moon-surfaced" island and home to the largest lizard living on earth, the fabulous and fierce Komodo dragon (*Varanus komodoensis*). Only here and on five neighboring islands do there be dragons. Dark gray and scaly with flabby necks, short snouts, and large mouths filled with small daggers, Komodo dragons are up to 10 feet in length, up to 500 pounds in weight, and up to no good when aggravated. Extraordinary athletes, they can easily run down the swiftest human runner and swim down the swiftest human swimmer. They can dig fast, climb fast, and eat fast, and their diet consists largely of meat: wild buffaloes, wild deer, wild pigs, wild goats, and wild-eyed humans dumb enough to get too near. A large part of their meals is carrion, and they've been known to raid graveyards, exhuming and devouring human corpses. They also eat each other, a habit that keeps baby Komodo dragons pretty much in the tops of trees for the first couple of years of life. Nearly deaf and nearly blind, these dragons can smell dinner up to 4 miles away with a favoring breeze.

Why You Die

Unless an impenetrable fence separates you from these giant lizards at feeding time, you are dead meat . . . or soon to be dead meat. Usually solitary, they team up at mealtime, when there's enough to go around. A dragon will charge you with great speed, aiming to take its first bite from your throat. It will hold you down with its forelegs and continue to rip off chunks of flesh, swallowing them whole. A team can easily polish off a whole human in 15 or 20 minutes.

To Live

You might be able to fight free, and fight you should. But even small nips from their notoriously germ-rich teeth will require attention from a medical specialist.

Moral: Good fences do not guarantee good neighbors.

KILLED BY KRAIT

God himself took a day to rest in, and
a good man's grave is his Sabbath.

JOHN DONNE, 1622

There are those who call it a relatively small serpent, with a length typically about 3 feet, but a few individuals have stretched out to almost 6 feet. It will probably be black, or maybe bluish black, and it will have 40 or so thin white rings around its cylindrical body. The rings may be faded or practically invisible on the head end. The flat head joins the body without anything resembling a neck. It will eat rats and mice, and frogs and lizards, but the common krait (*Bungarus cearuleus*) much prefers to dine on other snakes, including other kraits—which keeps it last on the list for any Snake Congeniality Award. Sometimes called the Indian krait, this snake lives everywhere you find jungle-like terrain in India and Sri Lanka. Many experts say kraits kill more humans every year than any other Indian serpent.

Kraits are seldom seen in daylight, but if you do find one in the glare of the sun, it may ball up and allow handling, now and then, without showing aggression. But handling, let it be said, is not highly recommended. At night, their time to be active, kraits will coil up, flatten out, and hide their heads when confronted. Be not fooled! They are now ready to strike.

Why You Die

Kraits seem to prefer not to bite, but if they do, they hold on grimly long enough to leave a large pool of venom in you. A krait's venom contains plenty of neurotoxins. Surprisingly, the bite itself may cause you little pain. But wait. Severe abdominal cramping is on the way, accompanied by spreading paralysis. Your breathing muscles are eventually paralyzed so you can't use them very well, so you suffocate to death.

To Live

About 8 out of 10 people bitten by kraits die without professional medical intervention. Find a medical professional to intervene. In the meantime, apply a pressure-immobilization bandage (see "Terrified by Taipan").

Moral: Do not fear the dark; fear
what the darkness hides.

16

MANHANDLED BY MAMBA

> All our life is but a going out to the
> place of execution, to death.
>
> JOHN DONNE, 1619

The mambas of Africa—black, green, western green, and Jameson's—closely related to cobras, are extremely agile and extremely fast, the fastest snakes on earth. They are also often extremely aggressive: If it is true that any snake will go out of its way to attack a human, this is the one, especially the black mamba (*Dendroaspis polylepis*). The most feared snake in Africa, black mambas grow to 14 feet in length with a width averaging between 3 and 4 inches. Among venomous snakes, only the king cobra grows larger (see "Clobbered by Cobra"). To add confusion, black mambas aren't black but gray or brownish gray, but the insides of their mouths are inky black. They prefer thick grass and dense brush, making a surprise meeting with a mamba likely and potentially deadly. They can climb trees almost as fast as they slither across the ground, and to add complications to your life, mambas are most dangerous when confronted with a moving target, at which they tend to strike thoughtlessly. When they lift their heads monstrously tall, taller than the tallest grass, it is the unusual human who will simply stand still and observe.

Why You Die

Among all snakes, the ill effects of being bitten usually appear most rapidly after mamba bites. Mambas are sometimes referred to as "three-step" snakes, meaning that you'll take three steps after the bite and keel over dead. It is not likely your death will occur that fast . . . four steps, maybe. Actually the venom, a neurotoxin, first causes, in most cases, difficulty swallowing, speaking, and seeing, followed by creeping paralysis that finally affects your respiratory system until you breathe no more. How fast this happens depends, in part, on how scared you are, but deaths have occurred in 15 minutes.

To Live

Find someone with the antivenin as soon as possible.

Moral: Watch your step.

17

MASSACRED BY MOCCASIN

> Could the Devil work my belief to
> imagine I could never die, I would
> not outlive that very thought.
>
> SIR THOMAS BROWNE, 1642

Being light of bone, snakes don't fossilize very well, so it's difficult to say when they first appeared in the grand scheme of things, somewhere probably between 8 and 20 million years ago. At some point along the evolutionary line, the pit vipers developed their unique, heat-sensitive facial pit, and many of them developed rattles. Copperheads and cottonmouth water moccasins, pit vipers both, do not grow rattles but are poisonous nonetheless. Especially dangerous is the water moccasin (genus *Agkistrodon*), rated by numerous experts as the third deadliest snake in the United States, causing more deaths than all other snakes except eastern and western diamondbacks (see "Reaped by Rattlesnake").

An inhabitant of shallow lakes, lazy streams, and swamps in the southeastern states and up to southern Illinois, the water moccasin grows 3 to 6 feet long, with a distinctly broad head leading its dull brownish-black body through life. White lines, sometimes easy to see, sometimes not, run back from both eyes. When it opens its mouth wide, the inside looks very white and "cottony." Known for their aggressiveness, moccasins, when threatened, tend to slither toward you instead of away.

Why You Die

You should feel pain and see swelling not long after either or both of the long fangs sink into your flesh. If you got it in a leg or arm, your whole extremity should look relatively disgusting within an hour, and certainly within a few hours, with blood-filled blebs forming near the bite site and black-and-blue colorations ascending toward your heart. You might feel tingling and numbness in your face and head. You might pull out of the experience in fairly healthy shape; or you might lose the arm or leg; or you might lose your blood pressure, go into shock and coma, and die as your blood loses its ability to support your life.

To Live

Run away very fast to avoid a bite. If bitten, try to stay calm (physically and emotionally), and remember that moccasins don't always envenomate when they bite (which should help you stay calm). Find a hospital with antivenin as soon as possible anyway.

> Moral: Keep your cotton-picking
> hands (and feet) to yourself.

18 PASSED ON BY PUFF ADDER

I know death is the fascinating snake
under the leaves, sliding and sliding.

MARY OLIVER, 1986

In the world of snakes, the names "adder" and "viper" are often used interchangeably (see "Eradicated by European Viper"). They, adders and vipers, are all members of the family Viperidae, and they are all venomous. The puff adder (*Bitis arietans*), a beefy snake, usually reaches about 40 inches in length but has been measured at 75 inches. Color patterns vary greatly depending on where you find the snake, but you'll probably see dark bands on the head, one between the eyes and one on the crown, and the head is always noticeably wider than the neck. Two things, however, make the puff adder worthy of special note: It is widespread on the continent of Africa, and it kills more humans in Africa than any other snake.

Their kill rate results partly from their broad range and partly from their habitually nasty disposition and partly from a venomous double whammy: really long fangs and a really potent poison. The scientific moniker *arietans* comes from the Latin for "striking violently." The violence of their strike sometimes kills small mammals before the venom has time to do its work. The power of the strike sinks the adder's fangs in deeply, followed by injection of a large amount of venom, usually 150–350 milligrams. An average adult human male can die from about 100 milligrams of puff adder venom. The adders curl into a tight S and hiss loudly when they feel threatened, and somehow the hissing gave rise to the name "puff."

Why You Die

To be fair, not all viper-bitten humans die. In fact, the survival rate for humans is around 85 percent. The venom, though, is cytotoxic, which means there will be lots of damage to your cells. Look for swelling and discoloration near the bite site, and blood blisters, and you may find it difficult to move a bitten arm or leg. You may permanently lose a bitten hand or foot. If your life ends, it will be due to uncontrollable external and, more significantly, internal bleeding.

To Live

You need to stay as calm as possible, move as little as possible, but get to a medical facility as soon as possible.

> Moral: Many things are possible,
> but not as many are probable.

19 REAPED BY RATTLESNAKE

Death's dark way must needs be
trodden once, however we pause.

HORACE, LET'S SAY 15 BCE

Living somewhere on earth today are approximately 2,700 kinds of snakes. Roughly 412 species are venomous enough to cause serious complications in the life of a human. In the United States members of two families of snakes have bites that could prove lethal: the Elapidae (see "Clobbered by Cobra" and "Corralled by Coral Snake") and the Crotalidae, the pit vipers, whose membership includes rattlesnakes. Not all the Crotalidae have rattles (see "Massacred by Moccasin"), but all rattlesnakes have rattles. Although experts continue to argue over the details, there seem to be about 36 species and subspecies of rattlesnakes rattling around in the United States. In addition to rattles, they all have a specialized venom injection system that works extremely well. It works like this: Venom is manufactured and stored in glands near the roots of two long, sharp, curved, hinged fangs. When the snake strikes, its mouth opens with the upper jaw almost 180 degrees from the lower jaw. The fangs spring 90 degrees down from the upper jaw and penetrate the victim. Venom is squirted down the hollow fangs and out a small orifice slightly above the point and in the front of the fang.

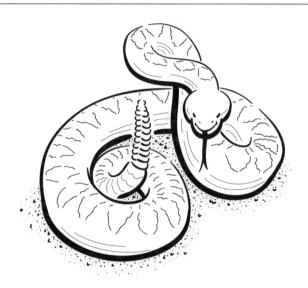

Diamondback rattlesnakes, the western and slightly larger eastern, cause most of the 10 to 15 deaths per year via snake in the United States, most often in people who try to handle the snakes or inadvertently step on one. Since rattlesnakes bite 7,000 to 8,000 humans in the United States every year, maybe a few less, maybe a few more, the chance that you'll be one to die is relatively small.

Why You Die

Although rattlesnakes do not envenomate with every bite, the venom causes immediate and intense pain and rapid swelling near the wound. In small creatures, say, a mouse, the venom is carried through the bloodstream and starts to dissolve the victim for easier digestion after the snake swallows the animal whole. In you the same process starts, but you won't totally dissolve. Just some of you dissolves, especially near where you got bit. Your red blood cells are broken down so they can no longer carry oxygen, and if enough of them are broken down, internal bleeding erupts, organs start to fail, cardiovascular shock rears its ugly head, and you bite the dust.

To Live

Stay calm. Running around and screaming after being bitten increases your chances of dying. Walk slowly, or better yet have someone carry you, to a hospital for the antivenin, which almost always works.

Moral: There's a lot to be said for staying calm.

TERRIFIED BY TAIPAN

Even Rome cannot grant us a
dispensation from death.

MOLIÈRE, 1665

Australia houses the world's greatest variety of the snakes
known collectively as elapids (family Elapidae), with at least
85 named kinds of these rather insolent venomous reptiles,
whose fangs are short and fixed in their upper jaws. Elapids,
which include the cobras, cause more human deaths than any
other snake family, and two Australian members are worthy
of special note.

If you were zipped into your dome tent with any snake, which one would give you the least chance of survival? When asked a similar question, one panel of experts unanimously voted the king cobra as "most dangerous" (see "Clobbered by Cobra"). Running second, but not far behind, was Australia's inland taipan (*Oxyuranus microlepidotus*), with venom reportedly the deadliest of all land snakes. A cousin, the coastal taipan (*Oxyuranus scutellatus*), growing to lengths of over 10 feet, is bigger, also very dangerous, but less venomous. These snakes vary in color, all typically unremarkable, such as gray, light brown, or cream. Scarce and rarely seen, quick to run when threatened, taipans counterattack when you try to pick them up. They suddenly turn ferocious, striking savagely and displaying a definite unwillingness to let go. Some victims, indeed, report having great difficulty removing the snake.

Why You Die

The neurotoxic venom causes a creeping paralysis that affects your ability to speak, swallow, and hold your eyes open. Your arms and legs will begin to weaken. If you survive, which happens, you'll probably have a lot of trouble healing the rotting muscles where the taipan bit. If you die, it will be preceded by increasingly difficult breathing until you no longer can. Some humans have survived the difficult-breathing stage only to die later when their kidneys failed.

To Live

You should immediately wrap a bitten arm or leg in an elastic bandage that extends from the fingers or toes all the way up the extremity, and you should splint the extremity. Then find a doctor who might have the antivenin.

Moral: Never pick up what you may not be able to put down.

21 TAKEN OUT BY TIGER SNAKE

It costs me never a stab nor squirm to tread
by chance upon a worm. Aha, my little dear,
I say, your clan will pay me back one day.

DOROTHY PARKER, 1928

Here we are not concerned with the harmless tiger snake of Africa, but the harmful tiger snake of Australia (family Elapidae, genus *Notechis*). A large snake, sometimes reaching 10 feet in length, it inhabits the southern parts of Down Under, including Tasmania and other islands off the southern coast. Colorwise the different species vary not only from region to region but also depending on the season of the year. You might see one green, brown, black, blue-black, gray, olive drab, or maybe another tint. But it will usually have tigerish stripes around its body of a different hue than the rest of the serpent. The belly will be lighter in color than the back.

Most often they slither quickly away from humans. But if a tiger snake feels trapped, it will curve up the front part of its body, flatten the rest of its body, slightly lift its head, and hiss. If you get too close, it will strike out swiftly and powerfully. Somewhere between 40 and 60 percent of those who are bitten die without first-class medical attention, making the tiger snake, to some experts, the deadliest Australian snake.

Why You Die

Tiger snake venom consists of neurotoxins (deadly to nerve tissue), myotoxins (causing muscle damage and paralysis), procoagulants (blood clotting disruptors), and hemolysins (things that kill red blood cells)—altogether a rather unappealing cocktail. Anticipate pain, then numbness and sweating, followed by spreading paralysis and increasing difficulty breathing. When you can't breathe at all, you die.

To Live

The recommended treatment for all Australian elapids, other than trying to stay still and calm (best wishes), is the pressure-immobilization bandage (see "Terrified by Taipan") and a dose of the very effective antivenin ASAP.

Moral: A tiger doesn't change his stripes.

DEATH BY

INSIDIOUS

INSECT

To be a member of the class Insecta, you need a three-part body (head, thorax, and abdomen), three pairs of legs, one pair of antennae, and compound eyes. A lot of creatures fit that description. At any given moment, the world's population of insects totals about 10 quintillion (a one followed by 19 zeros). In the United States alone you can find, if you're not busy with other stuff, approximately 91,000 species. Insects cause far more humans to die than all the other ways in this book combined.

22

ANNIHILATED BY ARMY ANTS

> One should die proudly when it is no
> longer possible to live proudly.
>
> FRIEDRICH NIETZSCHE, 1888

At least 150 species, and perhaps quite a few more, are known as "army ants," and like all ants, they are among the most fascinating creatures on earth, creating social structures among the most complex in the known universe. All army ants are true ants, of the family Formicidae, but unlike other ants, army ants are entirely nomadic, never building a nest but rather clumping together into a ball for egg laying. The clump may contain somewhere between 20 and 30 million individuals. When the urge to eat strikes, the colony migrates, carrying the larvae and taking hours to pass one specific point. Blind, or almost so, they follow a pheromone trail laid down by the leaders. At an invisible signal they crowd into a ball again while the queen lays her 25,000 or so eggs. Then they march again, and every living thing in their path must flee or perish.

Why You Die

Army ants literally tear their prey to shreds with powerful jaws. In South America the army ants tend to divide into two columns, forming a pincer movement to trap anything that moves and then devouring it. In Africa, however, the ants form fronts up to 2 miles wide and several miles long, pressing on relentlessly unless stopped by fire. They drive elephants mad, eat horses that were left tied, munch crocodiles caught away from water, and even send anteaters rushing away. If caught, you will be quickly and quietly overrun. Long before you go mad from the agony, you will die from shock or suffocate as they fill your nose and mouth.

To Live

Do not fall asleep on the ground in army ant country. Otherwise, since army ants are not fast, moving somewhere between 25 and 50 feet per hour on an average march, you should be able to outrun the colony, unless you're downed by a broken leg or staked out by someone who wishes you harm.

> Moral: Those who fear and run
> away live to run another day.

23

BOMBARDED BY BEE

It is nothing to die; it is frightful not to live.
VICTOR HUGO, 1862

When a honeybee gets riled up, it may deliver a sting with the sharp "needle" at the end of its abdominal section. Every stinger is attached to a venom sac. The venom causes immediate and sometimes frightful pain. When a swarm of honeybees gets riled up and attacks a human, the entire swarm delivers stings at an average rate of four stings per second. (*Note:* Killer bees, slowly migrating north from South America, are slightly smaller and darker than honeybees, but swarm far more aggressively and sting an average of 24 times per second.) If you run away, a wise move, you may have quite a few fiery wounds to deal with, but most humans survive just fine. The honeybees do not survive. The stingers are barbed; they rip out of the bee and stay in you, and the bee dies.

Bees, however, and their relatives in the order Hymenoptera (wasps, yellow jackets, hornets, fire ants), kill more humans in the United States every year than all the snakes, spiders, and scorpions combined. The reason: anaphylaxis.

Why You Die
Anaphylaxis is a severe allergic reaction brought on by a foreign protein getting into your blood. The protein in *Hymenoptera* venom causes allergic reactions in many humans.

If allergic, you may swell grossly soon after you're stung. But the death-dealing aspect of anaphylaxis, which usually occurs within minutes but can occur hours later, shows itself as extreme difficulty breathing and/or shock. Your face will be red and puffy, and your tongue will stick out as you desperately try to suck air in through your swollen airway. Although you won't know it, your blood pressure will drop dramatically. Within a very short time, you'll find yourself losing consciousness, and your spirit will buzz away forever.

To Live

If you are susceptible to anaphylaxis, you should know that the life-threatening reaction can be reversed, but only with an injection of epinephrine, sold by prescription.

Moral: Bee careful.

24

CONDEMNED BY CONENOSE BUG

Death is given in a kiss . . .
ROBERT LOUIS STEVENSON, 1878

Smooth and oval shaped, brownish in color, the conenose bug (or kissing bug, or assassin bug) is a Triatominae, taxonomically speaking, or a *vinchuca* to Spanish-speaking humans (meaning "one who lets himself fall down"). Less than an inch in length, the conenose bug has a long, narrow, cone-shaped head with two antennae and a proboscis that curves under. On the sides of the abdomen you might see narrow stripes of light yellow or red. It uses its two pairs of wings like a parachute to drop out of bushes and thatched roofs onto the faces of sleeping humans to feed on blood. This is most likely to happen somewhere in or between the southern United States and northern Argentina.

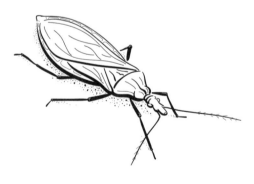

Once comfortable, most often near your mouth, the bug "kisses" with a scalpel-like extension of its proboscis and sucks your blood for about 20 minutes, ingesting many times its own weight. As it feeds it poops, and its poop contains a parasite, *Trypanosoma cruzi*, the cause of Chagas' disease. You rub your irritated wound after the bug leaves, you rub the parasite into you, and you get really sick.

Why You Die

After about one week you'll develop a hard, violet-hued bump where the bug bit. The parasites, clustered at the bump, begin to disperse throughout your body in your bloodstream. They invade your heart, brain, liver, and spleen. In children a severe brain infection may occur and lead to death. In adults the primary effect is on the heart, where lesions form that gradually reduce the effectiveness of your blood-pumping muscle. Some humans die in three months or so. Most humans survive initially to slowly succumb to the disease over the next 10 to 20 years.

To Live

Antiparasitic drugs are available to kill the parasites, and supportive care is recommended for other signs and symptoms of Chagas' disease.

Moral: A stolen kiss is often not worth it.

25

MURDERED BY MOSQUITO

We all labour against our own cure,
for death is the cure of all diseases.

SIR THOMAS BROWNE, 1642

For a long time, say 200 million years or thereabouts, the irritating whine of mosquitoes has plagued other living things on earth. Beginning life as larvae that wiggle almost invisibly in still water where mosquito eggs are laid, they progress to the pupal stage, frantically contorting back and forth like deranged commas, and finally to the insidious adult stage in which the females, who need blood to reproduce, go in search of a source. Both males and females can eat plant juice, but the males stick to their vegetarian diet. Females seek out anything with blood that they can stick their needle-tipped mouthparts into. With wings whirring at 600 beats per second, with eyes that see in virtually all directions at once, they primarily follow their sense of smell to heat, lactic acid, carbon dioxide, ammonia, and water vapor: signs of a warm-blooded animal.

Why You Die

Mosquitoes carry more germs that cause diseases than any other living creature in the entire known universe, and the females transmit the germs when they feed. They carry, for instance, the Zika virus. Although humans can die of Zika, death is rare. But a serious birth defect in babies born of moms infected with Zika is common. They also carry protozoa of the genus *Plasmodium*, including the four species that cause more than 200 million new cases of malaria per year (see "Mortified by Malaria"). They carry the germs for yellow fever, dengue fever (see "Doomed by Dengue"), and several forms of encephalitis, to name some of the most popular. In the United States the germs most likely to be found in mosquitoes cause West Nile virus (see "Wilted by West Nile"). Some experts state that approximately 700 million humans per year contract a mosquito-borne illness. This might explain why mosquitoes appear at the top of everyone's list of deadliest animals.

To Live

Use an insect repellent containing either DEET, Picaridin, oil of lemon eucalyptus, or IR3535, and follow the directions on the label. Limit your outdoor activities during prime mosquito-biting time: dawn and dusk. Wear long sleeves and long pants. Sleep under mosquito netting. Move to Antarctica or Iceland.

Moral: The only good skeeter is nowhere near where you are.

26

SCREWED BY SCREWWORM FLY

> Why, do you not know, then, that the origin of
> all human evils, and of baseness, and cowardice,
> is not death, but rather the fear of death?
>
> EPICTETUS, SECOND CENTURY CE

Many flies have the repugnant habit of laying their eggs in dead meat. The eggs hatch into maggots, which tenderize the dead meat with their excrement so they can eat it and eventually become adult flies. The screwworm fly (*Cochliomyia hominivorax* in the tropical New World, *Chrysomya bezziana* in the tropical Old World), about twice the size of a common housefly and blue-green to purplish black in color, has an even nastier habit.

Female screwworm flies lay their eggs in the wounds of living meat. Any wound will do, even a small scratch after a mosquito bite. If given free rein, she will lay up to about 500 eggs over a three- to five-day period. The eggs hatch in about 24 hours, sometimes as little as 12 hours, and the maggots, each about one-half inch at maturity, each looking somewhat like a small screw, eat their way with surprising rapidity into the living animal. In screwworm fly areas deaths among cows and sheep can be astounding in number. Eradicated in the United States, you can find these flies in Mexico and points south.

Why You Die

It will probably all start for you while you're asleep. The screwworm fly lays her eggs in, say, a little cut on your neck or shoulder or ankle. Death takes place when the maggots literally screw into your brain or lungs, which can take from a few days to a week.

To Live

Truthfully, your death via screwworm fly is unlikely unless for some reason you don't care for yourself. Or someone tied you to a tree in a fly-infested cow pasture in Costa Rica.

Moral: A swat in time saves lives.

27

TUCKED IN BY TSETSE FLY

> There is no God found stronger than
> death; and death is a sleep.
>
> ALGERNON CHARLES SWINBURNE, 1866

Although fossil evidence indicates it once buzzed around the prehistoric skies of North America, the brownish tsetse fly (family Glossinidae) now lives only in tropical Africa. It feeds in daylight, and it feeds on blood, and human blood is totally satisfying to the hungry fly. When driven by hunger, tsetse flies swarm viciously, bite through heavy clothing and rhino hide, and even attack the closed windows of vehicles. To humans the bite is briefly painful and itchy.

Born free of disease organisms, baby fly larvae feed off glands in mom for a while and then burrow into the ground to reappear 30 to 40 days later as full-blown flies. They leave the ground immediately in search of blood and drink up to three times their weight at a feeding. If the animal they drink from is infected with microscopic trypanosomes, which is often the case, the fly now carries these disease-causing organisms.

Why You Die

If you are bitten by a trypanosome-bearing tsetse, the single-celled parasites now enter your bloodstream. They multiply rapidly and start eating your own body's glucose. Bad things will start with a headache and fever and progress to increasing lethargy. You'll stumble your way through a period of anemia, seizures, and delirium before you slip into a coma, during which the "tryps" slowly take over. To the outside world you appear deeply asleep for a period of a few weeks to perhaps a few years. Death from sleeping sickness (trypanosomiasis)—which is related to Chagas' disease (see "Condemned by Conenose Bug")—involves complications in the functioning of your heart and/or nervous system.

To Live

There are drugs that will make you well.

Moral: Walk softly and carry a big swatter.

28

WOUNDED BY WASP

What is death?—a quiet of the heart?

LORD BYRON, 1816

A wasp is an insect of the order Hymenoptera but, and this may rank with the painfully obvious, it is not one of the bees (see "Bombarded by Bee") or one of the ants (see "Annihilated by Army Ant"), the other hymenopterans. Taxonomists delight in having identified and named more than 100,000 species of wasps, including all the yellow jackets and all the hornets. Even though you are used to the activity of social wasps, the ones that clump together in large numbers in a big shared nest, the worldwide majority of wasps are solitary creatures who build nests, if they do build one, for their immediate family only. Some solitary wasps are nonstingers. The ones who sting do so to kill prey and, therefore, do not uselessly sting a human. They will, of course, if they are threatened by, say, a swat from a hand. Social wasps sting in defense, and a single wasp can and will sting multiple times. Only female wasps have stingers, but the gender of the insect hardly matters when you are the target. And when one social wasp feels the need to be defensive, it releases a pheromone that angers all the stinger-packing members, a number that could be as high as 5,000, of the social colony. That's when you could be in trouble.

Why You Die

Wasp venom, injected by the stinger, breaks down local cell walls, causing the cells to send messages to your brain. The messages, as far as you are immediately concerned, are screams of pain. The pain can be intense but, thankfully, usually slacks off in a few minutes. Imagine, however, 100 stings, or 500 stings. Theoretically, you could die from a vast load of wasp venom. No one knows how many stings it would take. On the other hand, a large number of humans die every year from Hymenoptera stings due to anaphylactic shock (see "Bombarded by Bee"). Anaphylactic shock from bee and wasp stings kills more humans every year than any other death-by-venom category.

To Live

For one important thing, do not swat at a wasp. If you don't upset one wasp, you won't upset the colony. Remain still until it buzzes away, or until you can move quickly away from the little beastie. If you mess up and the colony swarms, run away at your maximum speed. If you're allergic (at risk of anaphylaxis), carry injectable epinephrine, a drug requiring a physician's prescription.

Moral: "Safety in numbers"
does not always apply.

DEATH BY MERCILESS MAMMAL

The class Mammalia includes animals that are warm-blooded, have hair (either a little or a lot), have a neocortex (part of the brain), and have (females only) mammary glands—and that means, for those who were unsure, humans are mammals. And so are whales, but they're in a different section of this book. Modern science currently recognizes 5,416 species of mammals. Most, but not all, have teeth; the ones in this section have teeth, some have claws, and none are afraid to use them.

29 | BRUTALIZED BY BEAVER

> All our knowledge merely helps us to die a more
> painful death than animals that know nothing.
>
> MAURICE MAETERLINCK, 1919

Ah, note the industrious beaver. It dams creeks and streams to form ponds, and then constructs a lodge in the pond in which to live and raise a family. It gnaws down surprisingly large trees during construction projects with its ever-growing teeth. A true wood addict, the beaver eats wood as well as chops it down. An excellent swimmer, its hind feet are webbed and its broad, flat tail is scaly. It makes a loud noise when it slaps its tail, when alarmed, on the surface of its pond. Beavers have their own genus (*Castor*), in which there are only two species: the North American beaver (*C. canadensis*) and the Eurasian beaver (*C. fiber*). The species are very closely related. Once they numbered an estimated 60 million or more, and now there are probably less than one-tenth that many. Beavers have not fared well in human vs. beaver conflicts. The world's second-largest rodent (behind the capybara), they grow throughout their lives and often reach more than 50 pounds in body weight. Appealing to watch, beavers are notoriously territorial and anger easily when threatened. Note, too, that they can kill you.

Why You Die

In search of an interesting way to die outdoors? Beaver attacks are admittedly rare, so that will make it interesting, but attacks are well documented and sometimes result in the last day of the human. If they can bite down a tree, there will surely be no problem in biting through your leg. When an artery is severed, your blood will flow abundantly. If you can't stop the blood loss, you will exsanguinate.

To Live

Give beavers plenty of room between them and you—and carry a tourniquet.

> Moral: You can be busy as a beaver
> but not busy with a beaver.

30

BESTED BY BENGAL TIGER

It takes so many years to learn that one is dead.

T. S. ELIOT, 1939

Bengal, the region, lies north of the Bay of Bengal, generally speaking, and includes parts of India and Bangladesh and lends its name to the world's most famous tiger, a feline that lives not only there but also in Nepal and Bhutan. Despite decreasing numbers, the Bengal tiger (*Panthera tigris tigris*) remains the most common tiger. It grows light orange or yellowish hair streaked with black or dark brown stripes. The stripes become black rings on the tail, and the belly is white. It may reach beyond 10 feet from nose to tip of tail and may weigh in at more than 700 pounds, and it boasts the longest teeth of all cats, teeth known to reach nearly 4 inches. The teeth, backed by powerful jaw muscles, are used to kill food—such as the deer, bison, and buffalo common to India and thereabouts. When their favored food runs low, Bengal tigers will attack animals much larger than themselves, with well-documented assaults on elephants and rhinos to their credit. And Bengals, unlike other tigers (see "Slain by Siberian Tiger"), sometimes develop a taste for human meat—which is not surprising when you remember that the densest tiger population is here jammed right up against the densest human population. Most Bengal tigers will take advantage, if they're hungry, of an opportunity to dine on a human, and a few become "man-eaters" and seek out leg of man even when other options are on the menu.

Why You Die

Tigers sneak as close as possible to their prey. A quick dash and a spring, and their teeth bury in your throat, and they hold on until you die, either from a broken neck, suffocation, or stark raving fear. They use their claws to help hold on in case you squirm. You will be dragged into a bushy spot, for a bit of privacy, and a hungry Bengal tiger may consume you entirely in one sitting.

To Live

Never run away! Do not turn your back. Tigers do not like to attack faces. Back away slowly and as calmly as possible. Do not crouch. Stand tall, raise your arms over your head, and attempt to look scary, but do not make eye contact. Eye contact seems to upset tigers. If you are a member of a group of humans, bunch together. If the tiger approaches closer, make loud noises, especially noises the tiger might find unusual—Handel's "Hallelujah Chorus," full volume, might work. If the tiger attacks anyway, you are having a really bad day.

> Moral: Having the eye of the tiger
> is sometimes a very bad idea.

31

BUFFALOED BY BISON

Let us endeavor so to live that when we come to die even the undertaker will be sorry.

MARK TWAIN, 1894

One of America's greatest losses, bison (*Bison bison*) once flowed like a vast, hairy sea, numbering in the millions, from the Alleghenies to the Sierra Nevada, from southern Texas to the Great Slave Lake in Canada, wandering in search of grass and water. Resembling Old World buffaloes, North American bison are a different species distinguished by massive, shaggy heads and shoulders and relatively small hindquarters. A mature bull may reach 6.5 feet in height and weigh in at more than a ton. Unmolested, they are a docile group (what remains of them), not given to harming humans.

Why You Die

Often viewed with pet-like affection by tourists in areas where they are protected, bison are sometimes pressed too closely by humans, arousing their sense of preservation, a survival instinct that has caused bison attacks in parks to outnumber bear attacks by more than four to one. Thundered into by the huge weight and muscle of a bison, you'll go somersaulting, coming to a stop battered, bruised, probably broken, and often dead. In addition, a horn or two will have gored you, in the butt if you're running away, in the abdomen if you face the charge. Your day will really fall apart if you happen to disturb an old bull whose herd follows nervously after him. After the subsequent trampling, depending on the size of the herd, what is left of you may be difficult to recognize and separate from the chips of dung that typically litter bison feeding grounds.

To Live
American bison rarely charge a human unless approached to within 25 feet.

Moral: Don't be a chip off the old bison.

32

BUTCHERED BY BLACK BEAR

Death is what men want when the anguish
of living is more than they can bear.

EURIPIDES, 425 BCE

As far as bears go, black bears (*Ursus americanus*) do not grow very large, maybe 6 feet and 500 pounds in an extreme case, but they range over a vast area, from northern Alaska to Mexico, Florida to California, Maine to Washington State. In color, too, they can range widely: black, cinnamon, blond, blue, brown, almost white. Omnivorous and shy and very strong, they can also be short-tempered. Black bears in many areas have grown quite used to having humans around and, as a result, are turning more and more to humans as a food source. Especially dangerous are older, weaker black bears that can catch and kill little other than a puny, slow-moving man or woman. And to a bear all men and women are puny and slow-moving. As a matter of record, black bears have killed and eaten more humans than grizzly bears have (see "Gutted by Grizzly").

Attracted by thoughts of easy pickings, black bears in recent years have torn through the door of a travel home to consume the contents, particularly the human resident; climbed onto the roof of a cabin to knock off and eat the human occupant; and devoured the arms off of a hiker before leaving her for dead. When you consider the number of black bears and the number of humans, however, bear attacks are still relatively rare.

Why You Die

When a black bear does attack a human, it does not have any playful intent. The bear is either hungry or protective of its young. If it's hungry, you are food. These bears seldom even bother to kill you first. They just grab hold and start munching. You may have the exceedingly rare opportunity to feel yourself being ripped apart and watch the meal, which is you, in progress. You will not usually have much time to watch.

To Live

Those wishing to not be bear food report success from returning the bear's attack, beating the animal on the head and face with anything available, including fists, and otherwise resisting consumption as long as strength allows.

Moral: Stand up and fight for your rights.

33

BLASTED BY BUFFALO

Everything on earth fades fast, Death will take us all at last, that's a truth we know won't pass.

GEORG BÜCHNER, 1836

True buffaloes should not be confused with American bison (see "Buffaloed by Bison") and are, beyond a shadow of the bloodiest doubt, the most potentially lethal of all ungulates. In all of Africa the great buffalo (*Syncerus caffer*) is considered by many experts to surpass all the other dangerous animals (the lion, leopard, elephant, hippo, and rhino) in dangerousness.

Though relatively placid if undisturbed, buffaloes are cunning and easily upset, and notoriously antagonistic toward humans if wounded, cornered, or surprised by your appearance in tall, dense grass. With heavy, sharp-tipped horns that emerge from the middle of their iron-plate-like skulls, buffaloes have been known to have bullets bounce off them while they dodge hunters and circle around to attack from behind. Their huge bulk is no deterrent to their alarming speed. They aim for a gouge with the horns.

Why You Die

Once hooked by the horns, you'll be tossed in the air, possibly to a height of 10 feet or more. On the ground, prostrate and bleeding, you have only begun to die. A buffalo will charge

Death by Merciless Mammal

back to spear you again. But this time it'll toss its head angrily and mightily from side to side until you have been shredded. So irate is the irate buffalo that one well-documented account reports a human who climbed a short tree to escape but could not get his feet above the bull's horns. The buffalo repeatedly slashed the feet until the poor guy bled to death. He was found hanging in the tree, drained of blood. Now that's interesting!

To Live
Avoid really tall grass, and do not ever wound, corner, or surprise a buffalo.

Moral: The horns of a dilemma can be fatal.

34

CHEWED BY CAMEL

> Death is a camel that lies down at every door.
>
> PERSIAN PROVERB

All the hoofed animals of the world are collectively known as ungulates. They are divided into two orders depending on whether they have an odd number of toes (such as horses, rhinoceroses, and tapirs) or an even number of toes (such as pigs, cows, sheep, goats, deer, llamas, and camels). Though ungulates are generally docile, notable exceptions exist (see "Blasted by Buffalo"). To the exceptions you may also add, now and then, camels.

The Arabian camel, *Camelus dromedarius*, has one hump and is used as a beast of burden in hot, sandy regions such as Arabia and parts of Africa. The Bactrian camel, *Camelus bactrianus*, has two humps and is seen most often in cooler, rockier areas such as northern Asia.

Camels are known around the world for their ability to store large amounts of water and go for long days and long miles without refreshment. They are less known for but just as liable to be foul of temper. As a burden bearer, they hate to be overloaded, and they will secretly hold intense hatred for an abusive handler, biding their time and attacking when least expected. Sometimes they attack for no known reason.

Why You Die

Camels attack with their teeth. Unlike most herbivores, they have canine teeth that have been known to sever a human limb. If your limb doesn't sever, they'll lift their heads up and back, flipping you around with enough force to literally break your neck. If that doesn't work, and they get you on the ground, they'll keep biting until you bleed to death. They have also been known to kick during an attack, and even to lie down on the human they find offensive. One hump or two? Who cares? Your screams will not bother them in the least.

To Live

Run away, preferably toward shelter, such as a building or vehicle. If bitten, fight back.

Moral: Don't be a burden to others.

CARVED UP BY CANNIBAL

Life is a great surprise. I do not see why
death should not be an even greater one.

VLADIMIR NABOKOV, 1962

Nothing in the wildest imagination has come near to ending as many human (*Homo sapiens*) lives as other humans: Note such things as homicides, wars, inquisitions. Over the years a surprising number of those human deaths have been followed by feasts in which the dead humans were dinner for fellow humans. After their hearts had been torn out on altars, sacrificed men and women regularly became a meal for the Aztecs, the meat usually stewed with tomatoes and peppers. The Senga country of Africa has a long history of cannibalism dating back well before the first historians started making notes on African eating habits. Whether or not they threw living missionaries into pots of boiling water remains a moot point, unless you were one of the missionaries. When Columbus "discovered" America, he was warned to stay off several islands of the Indies where the Carib Indians were very fond of roasting and consuming invited and uninvited "guests." The word *barbecue*, in fact, is a Spanish corruption of the Indian word for their roasting device. Several lost-in-the-wilderness incidents have become famous because the survivors ate the dead.

Even more startling is the number of cannibals who still today break their fasts on leg of man or arm of woman. This is mostly done in areas where McDonald's and microwaves do not exist, and mostly done by one primitive tribe to another whose flavor has found favor. If you wandered in at mealtime, however, there's no reason to think you might be spared.

Why You Die

Fine chefs, it seems, will always butcher you first and add a few condiments, so at least you won't have to wait for the water to boil.

To Live

Put up a good fight.

> Moral: Better to know who you're having for dinner than who's having you.

36 CORNERED BY CAPE HUNTING DOGS

> It hath often been said, that it is not
> death, but dying, which is terrible.
>
> HENRY FIELDING, 1751

Domestic dogs occasionally show up in the news as killers and, rarely, devourers of owners or, more often, of neighbors or postal service workers. Dobermans and pit bulls figure in many of these accounts. Their attacks are often indoors or at least in the backyard, and they really don't qualify, even though they are interesting, as outdoor deaths. But domestic dogs have close relatives in the wild outdoors: true wild dogs, family Canidae, which include the small, spotted, big-eared Cape hunting dogs (*Lycaon pictus*), also known as African wild dogs.

Traveling in packs of 5 to 50, these dogs are extremely opportunistic feeders—if they get the opportunity, they feed. Being relatively keen of intelligence, wild dogs fear humans and shun them most of the time. A lone human, however, to a hungry pack might well become dinner.

Why You Die

Working as a well-coordinated team, wild dogs will surround you. A rush by one dog can be turned with a kick or a blow to its nose with a stick or rock. But while you're striking at dog one, dog two runs in to tear out one of your leg muscles with sharp teeth powered by crushing strength. Once you're on the ground, it's all over in a matter of seconds: A half-dozen dogs are savaging your arms and legs while one brute rips out your throat. For what it's worth, in the spirit of the finest environmentalists, none of you will go to waste.

To Live

While in wild dog country, travel in a pack of humans.

Moral: There's safety and danger in numbers.

37

CONSUMED BY COUGAR

Death is stronger than all the governments
because the governments are men
and men die and then death laughs:
now you see 'em, now you don't.

CARL SANDBURG, 1950

Mountain lion, puma, panther, catamount, or cougar: All the names point to one animal, *Felis concolor*, the largest wild cat of the United States, a feline that might reach a weight of 200 pounds. While they once roamed with quiet dignity from southern Canada to the tip of South America, in forest and in field, cougars now are seen rarely outside the wildest areas of the western United States except for very rare sightings in the swamps of Georgia and Florida. Still, no cat on earth has adapted to as broad a range of latitudes or habitats as the cougar.

No doubt exists whatsoever that mountain lions would greatly prefer never to see a human being. As their habitats become increasingly cluttered with humans, however, a simultaneous and slight increase in cats viewing humans as food has naturally occurred.

A cougar may also attack if cornered, announcing the attack by laying its ears back, snarling, and twitching its tail. As with all cats, cougars may be attracted to you by simple curiosity, but become frightened and kill.

Why You Die

Cougars are powerful, with long, sharp claws and long, sharp teeth. Like most predators, they would much rather you not know they were coming in for a kill. A slinking up, a sudden pounce, teeth closing over your neck, and you're dragged to the ground, perhaps never knowing what broke your neck.

To Live

Face an approaching cougar. Do not run. Try to appear fierce and unappetizing. Pick up a rock, stick, or other weapon. If it keeps coming, yell, throw things, and show your teeth. If it still keeps coming, charge the cougar, striking at its face but staying out of claw range. If it attacks, fight back with all your strength, aiming your blows at the eyes, nose, and ears.

Moral: Curiosity kills more than cats.

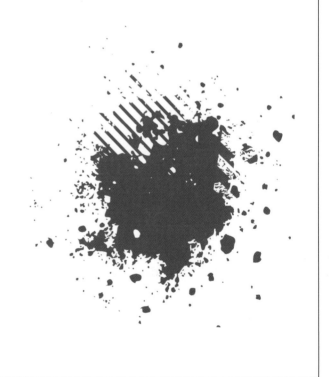

38

ELIMINATED BY ELEPHANT

Dust thou art, and unto dust thou shalt return.
GENESIS 3:19

Once more than 350 kinds of elephants roamed with relative tranquility over the face of the earth, not bothered by much, not bothering much. Today only two species remain: the African elephant and the Asiatic or Indian elephant. Entirely vegetarian, they daily consume vast quantities of grasses and leaves, fruits, and small twigs, as much as 400 pounds per 24 hours, which they grind with four large teeth before swallowing. Social by nature, they live and move in herds with strong family ties, broken only by adult bulls that leave the herd of cows and calves to lead solitary lives, returning for brief visits during the mating season.

An adult male African elephant (*Loxodonta africana*) may stand above 10 feet at the shoulder and weigh in at more than six tons. His tusks, elongated incisor teeth, grow his whole life and have been known to reach 10 feet in length and 230 pounds each in weight. He can run at better than 20 miles per hour for long periods of time. Though gentle by nature, he can be pushed beyond the endurance of his massive patience. An enraged bull elephant, African or Indian—and females get enraged sometimes, too—will not be deterred from utterly ensuring you are dead.

Death by Merciless Mammal

Why You Die

An elephant will taste the you-scented air with its trunk, swinging it from side to side and then straight out toward you while its ears spread wide to guide every tiny sound you make into its ear canals. Its barely useful eyes will glisten wetly as it dances an awkward shuffle, rolling its weight from side to side. Before you realize it has started to charge, dust billows around its chest and front legs, and all appearance of awkwardness suddenly dissolves into forward motion accompanied by a shrill and heart-stopping blast of sound. If your heart starts again and fear allows you to run, your dash will cover little ground before the elephant's trunk wraps around your waist and you are lifted high over the animal's head. (*Note:* If a male happens to spear you with a tusk, it will be an accident, but he won't care.) The thump of your body smashing with terrific force onto the ground will probably end all interest you have in your own death, but your ruin has only begun. Pressing you firmly into the soil, the elephant will use its trunk to tear you raggedly into approximately two halves. Each half will be systematically stomped until no bone remains unbroken. At last satisfied, the elephant will raise its trunk in a final trumpet of glorious victory. Later you will easily assume the shape of whatever vessel is chosen to carry away the pulp that was once a human being.

To Live

If charged, throw away a hat or shirt to distract the elephant. If you can, climb a very stout tree. If all else fails, try standing still. Elephants will sometimes abandon a charge when the source of their agitation is not moving.

Moral: The bigger they are, the harder you fall.

39

GRABBED BY GORILLA

Any man's death diminishes me, because I am involved in mankind; and therefore never send to know for whom the bell tolls; it tolls for thee.

JOHN DONNE, 1624

Members of the group called "great apes" are divided into chimpanzees (genus *Pan*), orangutans (*Pongo*), and the greatest of all, gorillas (*Gorilla*). Both mountain and lowland gorillas are found only in equatorial Africa, where although they are shorter than most men and women, they grow to outweigh humans by several hundred pounds, with arm spans that may exceed 9 feet. Gorillas have stupendous strength and extraordinary intelligence, but their ability to maim and ruin is more than matched by their quiet and gentle spirits. Though able to destroy just about anything, gorillas are satisfied with a ferocious glare, a mighty bellow, and a few thumps on their massive chests. They will charge you in a most realistic fashion, but physical contact with humans ranks among the rarest of incidents. Gorillas live most of their lives with four extremities on the ground, their two feet and the knuckles of their two hands. They perform their bluff charges that way, and almost everything so confronted turns and runs. You'll have to work very hard if you want to be killed by a gorilla.

Why You Die

Should you wade in with fists flying, you might be able gener-
ate a devastating sideways swat or a tremendous bite from a
gorilla's large mouth, associated with giant teeth and powerful jaw muscles. The gorilla will then tend to withdraw. If you
are conscious and able, you could counterattack the gorilla's
counter of your attack, and possibly get annihilated, a fate
you would infinitely deserve.

To Live

Be more like a gorilla.

Moral: Leave well enough alone.

40

GUTTED BY GRIZZLY

Death is not anything . . . It's the absence
of presence, nothing more . . . the
endless time of never coming back . . .
a gap you can't see, and when the wind
blows through it, it makes no sound.

TOM STOPPARD, 1967

For thousands of years the great brown bears ruled North America from the Bering Strait to northern Mexico. Now they hide in Alaska and western Canada and in a few wilderness areas of the western United States, subdued by the gun, the fear, and the greed of humans.

Growing to over 1,000 pounds in weight, inland brown bears, the grizzlies (*Ursus arctos horribilis*), are immense mounds of muscle that can run at better than 35 miles an hour. A large hump on their shoulders distinguishes the "griz" from all other bears. They possess huge feet with non-retractable claws and huge omnivorous appetites appeased on a daily basis by about 80 percent vegetables and fruit. The other 20 percent of their diet is meat.

Grizzly bears attack humans seldom and most often because they feel threatened. But on rare occasions a bear will attack for no apparent reason except perhaps a quick snack. Although they appear most ferocious in paintings where the artist depicts them on their hind feet swiping powerfully at some poor human soul, grizzly bears spend most of their lives on four feet, and they charge on four feet. Their claws are primarily for gathering food and secondarily for taking swipes at things. Their teeth are for killing and tearing off hunks of meat for consumption.

Why You Die

The best way to encourage a grizzly bear to attack is to run. Giving chase is one of their chief sources of entertainment. They can run fast for a long time. As soon as you get caught, remember that they also enjoy wrestling, possibly because they always win. Fighting back encourages the bear to fight.

It will cheat, biting relentlessly, especially your head and neck. Once you're dead, the bear may or may not eat you, depending on its hunger. If it decides to eat, it will likely start with your guts, the most tender and juicy part of you. Either way, you lose.

To Live

Do not run. Stand tall, and face the bear. It may bluff charge and then walk away. If it attacks, playing dead often, but not always, discourages the grizzly bear, which then loses interest in you. Lie on your face with your arms protecting your head and neck. If the bear rolls you over, keep rolling until you are face down again. Be sure the bear is long gone before you stand.

Moral: If there's no chance you'll win, don't play.

41

HARASSED BY HIPPOPOTAMUS

It is death that is the guide of our life,
and our life has no goal but death.

MAURICE MAETERLINCK, 1896

Once they wobbled fatly over the entire continent of Africa, but now hippopotamuses, "river horses," stake out their territories in relatively small regions in shallow rivers with open grassland nearby. They are prevalent, for instance, in the Zambezi River of Zimbabwe.

They stick to the water during the day, nibbling water plants, and come out at night to graze on land plants, primarily grass. Hippos (*Hippopotamus amphibious*) require an average of between 50 and 90 pounds of food per day to sustain their 3,000- to 9,000-pound bodies—but individuals may consume 150 pounds of grass in a day. Hippos have also been reported to occasionally eat meat. Although they clump together in sociable herds, the encroachment of any human into their territory typically causes an attack by a dominant male or a nursing mother. Hippos may be the most dangerous animals in Africa, killing more humans every year than all the lions, elephants, and buffaloes combined.

In the water they are especially aggressive, easily "swimming" down any human and chomping small boats in half. They actually swim rather poorly and sink to the bottom immediately when the water deepens over their heads. They

Death by Merciless Mammal

run along the bottom of rivers, staying underwater for up to five minutes. On land they are capable of reaching speeds of 45 miles per hour when aroused.

Why You Die

A hippo yawns to warn you. Inside that monstrously gaping mouth are sharp canine teeth driven by powerful jaw muscles that can snap shut with more than 2,000 pounds of pressure. One chomp with no swallowing will usually satisfy the hippo, and easily satisfies the coroner who is required to list your cause of death.

To Live

In water give hippos a very wide berth. On land you cannot outrun a determined hippo, but running is advised since they might lose interest.

Moral: The wise heed warnings.

42

HOUNDED BY HYENA

> Life does not cease to be funny when people die any more than it ceases to be serious when people laugh.
>
> GEORGE BERNARD SHAW, 1913

Frequently thought of as cowards slinking just outside the light of your campfire, eaters of carrion whose demented laughs pierce the darkest African nights, hyenas are relatively intelligent, strict meat eaters, and, even though they do scavenge, capable of aggressive attacks, singly and in teams, on very-much-alive humans.

With wide grins and backs that slant noticeably toward the rear, hyenas (collectively called Hyaenidae) appear like canines designed by a committee of politicians but actually have more attributes of cats than dogs. Equipped with some of the most powerful jaws in the animal kingdom, hyenas can snap bones that defy the teeth of more formidable-looking mammals. Their range, once throughout most of Europe, Asia, and Africa, is now limited to parts of Africa, India, and the Near East.

Why You Die

Hyenas have nasty dining habits that include a marked tendency to eat and run: They'll rush up to you while you doze unprotected, rip off a significant portion of your face (their favorite target), and dash into the bush while still swallowing. If you are small enough, a hyena will grab an arm or leg and bound away with you in tow. Your screams will linger in the night air and bear no resemblance to a laugh.

To Live
Never deeply committed to munching humans, hyenas are extremely dedicated to opportunity eating, and thus are creatures you should resist trusting. They will tend to abandon you as a meal if you are adequately aggressive.

Moral: He who laughs last laughs best.

43

JOLTED BY JAGUAR

Death eats up all things, both the
young lamb and the old sheep.

CERVANTES, AROUND 1605

Possibly entirely gone now from the extreme southwestern United States, the jaguar (*Panthera onca*) holds on tenaciously as the only living member of the *Panthera* genus in the Western Hemisphere. You can find them in Mexico and lands south. Yellowish in color, with a much darker animal showing up now and then, they are littered with dark splotches. Their bellies, however, are a spotless white. Sizewise, no cats on earth grow larger except lions and tigers. In southern Brazil, jaguars have tipped a scale to well over 300 pounds. From the nose to the base of the tail, individuals have exceeded 6 feet, but they are typically shorter. And speaking of short, for their size their legs are not very long. Short legs help them slink along near the ground as they sneak up on prey, but they also are amazingly adept at climbing tall trees and swimming wide rivers. Amazing, too, is the power of their bite. A hungry jaguar will crack open a turtle's shell to obtain the morsels within, something lions and tigers cannot do—or at least chose not to do. No jaguar has ever been known to become a man-eater—but on rare occasions jaguars have attacked and brutally killed humans.

Why You Die

While most cats go for the neck of their prey, jaguars like to bite the skull, crushing it and the brain. This will most likely happen to you in Brazil, where the cats are larger, but bitten-to-death-by-jaguar human brains show up from time to time in more northern locales.

To Live

If the jaguar misses your skull, the teeth will most likely be buried in your shoulder. Now would be a good time to fight back, striking at the eyes and nose. As with other large cats, confrontations that have yet to involve a bite will work best for you if stand tall, raise your arms, make loud noises, and back away (see "Bested by Bengal Tiger"). Keep facing the jaguar, and never run. You could also try wearing a football helmet.

Moral: Never turn your back on a snarl.

44

LEAPED ON BY LEOPARD

It is better that we live ever so
miserably than die in glory.

EURIPIDES, 405 BCE

Even though these cats are divided into at least 15 "races" that range from southern Africa north into Russia, from Malaysia to Israel, from below sea level to 18,000 feet, they are all basically the leopard (*Panthera pardus*), one of if not the most widely distributed large mammal on earth. Among all the cats of the world that regularly kill and consume humans, the leopard holds a special place. Smallest of the man-eaters, reaching maybe 120 pounds, the leopard is by weight the most powerful, able to drag a 150-pound man 4 miles after the kill, and despite its size, the most intelligent. Leopards, say the experts, know what you're thinking. With no other cat is the hunter more likely to become the hunted . . . and the devoured. Individual leopards that have become dedicated to man-eating have ended the lives of as many as 400 men, women, and children.

Why You Die
Extraordinarily keen of night sight, leopards sneak up in utter silence to leap, always, for the throat of their victim, be it antelope, buffalo, or you. From behind, your neck will most likely be broken by the powerful bite. From the front your

windpipe will be torn out, resulting in death by suffocation. Either way, four long canines are driven in faster than a carpenter could drive in nails with a nail gun. And leopards have the extremely brutal habit of ripping repeatedly with their hind claws, shredding with needle-tipped daggers until your guts are strewn along the ground, a problem with which you will have no concern since you'll be close enough to death by then not to care.

To Live
Avoid darkness in the land of the leopard, primarily a nocturnal hunter. As with all cats, you may have a chance to fight a leopard off—if you see it coming.

> **Moral:** Discretion is the better part
> of remaining in one piece.

45

LUNCHED ON BY LION

To die is to leave off dying and
do the thing once for all.

SAMUEL BUTLER, 1902 OR THEREABOUTS

The lion (*Panthera leo*) once roamed with kingly or queenly mien over all of Africa except the densest forest and highest mountains and well north into Europe and throughout the Near East. Now it is an animal almost exclusively of the open bush and savanna, the great grasslands of Africa, never entering the jungle, with remnant populations in parts of Asia and India. Weighing in at 200 to 400 pounds (or sometimes more) and able to leap 20 feet or more in a single bound, *P. leo* is not the largest or most powerful cat, an honor held by the Siberian tiger, a close relative (see "Slain by Siberian Tiger"). Female lions do most of the day-to-day hunting and killing, typically

Death by Merciless Mammal

at dawn, dusk, and night, singling out a slow, weak individual from a herd. Aside from the occasional man-eater with an odd predilection for humans, almost always a lone male, lions prefer a juicy antelope or a toothsome wildebeest, but they have few reservations about lunching on a bipedal primate when the menu is limited. With little stamina, lions are relegated to one short burst of astounding speed. That's usually all it takes.

Why You Die

A dash and a leap, and the lion makes contact with your quivering flesh. A staggering blow from a forepaw of remarkable strength will be quickly followed by the sinking of long teeth into your neck. One bite and your neck snaps, and whatever interest you had in life fades faster than a speeding bullet. Your last movement will be a couple of involuntary and convulsive kicks. One lion will eat up to 60 pounds at one sitting. If the pride shares you, tearing off great hunks for a noisy gulp, you'll be no more than a single fast-food meal.

To Live

If a lion charges, run toward it. It is, say the experts, your best chance of stopping the charge. If that fails, fight back, while screaming (which usually comes naturally) to confuse the lion—although it might be futile.

> **Moral:** In lion country travel in the middle of herds of slower, weaker humans.

46

MASTICATED BY MONGOOSE

> The tongues of dying men enforce
> attention like deep harmony.
>
> WILLIAM SHAKESPEARE, 1595

The name Rikki-tikki-tavi will ring a bell of remembrance for millions of humans because they read Rudyard Kipling's *The Jungle Book*, or they heard someone talking about the most famous of all mongoose vs. cobra encounters—or they saw the animated version of the story. Rikki is indeed a mongoose, and so too Timon of *The Lion King*, although Timon and his close kin are usually called meerkats. They are 2 of 34 currently identified members of the family Herpestidae. Their long weasel-like faces, small ears, and short legs make you think weasel, but they are all feliforms, cat-like carnivores. Widespread in Africa, they are also common in southern Asia, and you may see one on several islands, including Fiji and Puerto Rico. Depending on species, they range in weight from the 11-ounce dwarf mongoose to the 11-pound white-tailed mongoose. Often a solid dark brown, or light brown, or gray, they can be yellowish or banded in light and dark stripes. And it is very true that their lightning-fast reflexes allow them to successfully attack and kill very poisonous snakes. As carnivores, their diet includes lots of rodents, birds, lizards, snakes, eggs, and meat that has been lying around dead for a while. They have been well documented, though rarely, to kill and partially devour a human.

Why You Die
In fairness to mongooses, they almost always prefer to run away from humans. But in days of drought and, therefore, short supplies of food for animals such as mongooses, these furry little creatures will attack a small human, usually a small child. They bite viciously, the neck when they can reach it, and the human bleeds to death. Mongooses also are susceptible to rabies (see "Ravaged by Rabies"), and death from a rabid mongoose has occurred.

To Live
As common sense suggests, give all mongooses plenty of room, especially if you are little. If you do get bitten, wash the wound immediately and aggressively with soap and water for, say, 10 minutes. Then find a doctor and tell your tale.

Moral: It's not how big you are;
it's how hungry you are.

47

MESSED UP BY MOOSE

Death is a thing of grandeur . . . It is
a rearrangement of the world.

ANTOINE DE SAINT-EXUPÉRY, 1942

Deer are ubiquitous and come in a great variety, tiny to hulking, around the world. Of all the large mammals, they are usually the last to flee the encroachment of human development, indicating that they are either very brave, very stubborn, or not very smart. Hunted heavily in most areas, however, deer have grown reasonably afraid of humans and retire readily when approached . . . most of the time.

Sharp of hoof, with a weight that might reach beyond 1,500 pounds, with antlers that may spread to 8 feet across, moose (genus *Alces*) are the largest members of the deer family and particularly easy to offend, especially in the season of the rut, when bulls establish their harems and charge any intruder at the slightest provocation. Moose wounded by careless hunters regularly attempt to kill the hunter. On national parkland, where tourists tend to think of wild animals as not so wild, irate moose have been known to attack automobiles and sink small boats (moose spend a lot of their days in water), and end human lives.

Why You Die

Lowered head, flaring nostrils, flattened ears, and bristling hair indicate a moose is upset. Head down and hooves thundering across the wilderness, a charging moose is an impressive spectacle. It'll lead with an antler, and you'll go flying with ripped flesh and crushed bone. Once you're subdued, moose seldom hesitate to use their hooves for a few final tromps, just to make sure you understand their dislike of your trespass. You do not need to die to satisfy moose. They'll walk away while you're still breathing. But dead or alive, you're going to be a mess.

To Live

Never, ever approach a moose, even if it appears docile. If attacked anyway, put a tree or rock between you and the moose. It may take a while, but it will eventually tire of the game of "kill the intruder."

Moral: Neatness counts.

48

PULVERIZED BY POLAR BEAR

Death takes us piecemeal, not at a gulp.
SENECA, FIRST CENTURY CE

Bears appear worldwide, one of the most broadly distributed mammals on the face of the planet, and they are all relatively similar. But only the polar bear (*Ursus maritimus*) is circumpolar, found in every nation that shares the Arctic Circle, and only the polar bear lives entirely on meat. These fluffy white or yellowish-white bears are perfectly adapted to the typically white landscapes across which they roam. And being the largest land carnivore on earth (up to 10 feet long and 1,600 pounds) and an inhabitant of harsh environments where humans seldom intrude, the polar bear has little fear of humans and no hesitation about feasting on a human if hunger drives it to consume something less appetizing than a fat seal (preferably the skin, blubber, and organs). Polar bears can sniff out blubber, seal or human, from 20 miles away. They may occasionally cough or roar, but most of their lives are quiet, and quietly they sneak up on their prey for a quick pounce. If necessary, but not as their first choice, they can run up to 25 miles per hour to overtake their next meal. They swim well enough to catch sea birds and have even been known to overturn a small boat in order to munch on a succulent Inuit who happened to be paddling by.

Death by Merciless Mammal

Why You Die

Polar bear attacks on humans fall into two general categories: (1) You surprise a bear, usually a mother bear with young, and you receive a powerful but seldom fatal swat to remind you to stay away. (2) You are hunted as food, and found; and your death, by claw and fang, is almost instantaneous—after which you are rapidly torn into bite-size pieces and consumed.

To Live

Travel in large groups, never alone; make lots of human-sounding noises; and try to smell skinny.

Moral: Always hike with someone
who runs slower than you.

49

WRECKED BY RHINOCEROS

> The last act is tragic, however happy all the rest of the play is; at the last a little earth is thrown upon our head, and that is the end for ever.
>
> BLAISE PASCAL, 1670

Descended from the largest land mammal ever to roam the earth, a creature that was at least 18 feet at the shoulder, rhinoceroses are kin to horses but have grown very thick hides and a horn or two on their noses. Though they once numbered in the hundreds of thousands, currently the world enjoys fewer rhinos than American bison. Their name comes from two Greek words *rhinokeros*, meaning "nose horn," and five species inhabit today's earth: Indian rhinos, Javan rhinos, Sumatran or "hairy" rhinos, white rhinos, and black rhinos. All are nearsighted and short-tempered, keen of smell, and keen on trampling anything that lies in their path when they suddenly erupt into high-speed charges. Africa's black rhino (*Diceros bicornis*) is rated the greatest opportunity for death.

The reaction of rhinos to an unusual sound (the click of a camera, the rustle of grass) or smell (you) is to charge over to find out what's going on. They have been known to charge at full speed, about 35 miles per hour, into cars, buses, even trains. A myth surrounding a rhino's charge is that you can wait until the last moment and quickly sidestep it. Not so!

Death by Merciless Mammal

Rhinos in full charge can turn on a dime and give five cents change, and they have the nasty habit of hooking right and left with their horns when they get within striking range. Unless you're Tarzan, it won't work.

Why You Die

The result of being caught by a rhino's charge is that you're hooked on the horn and tossed 12 feet or so into the air. If the rhino misses with the horn, it will probably plow you underground beneath its thundering feet. Either way, or both ways at once, you tend to be quite dead and messy by the time a rhinoceros figures out you are no particular threat.

To Live

If you discover you can't outrun a rhino, try falling flat and lying still. Rhinos have lost interest in fleeing victims when they suddenly stopped fleeing.

Moral: Great distances make good neighbors.

50

SAVAGED BY SEAL

The most rational cure after all for the inordinate fear of death is to set a just value on life.

WILLIAM HAZLITT, 1821

Of the 47 kinds of pinnipeds (see "Wasted by Walrus") that swim the earth's waters with their mermaid-like tails, none ranks as fiercer of aspect when confronted with a human than the leopard seal (*Hydrurga leptonyx*). Residents of difficult-to-access areas of the Antarctic and sub-Antarctic, leopard seal males grow to 10 feet and 600-plus pounds while the females may reach 12 feet and 1,000 pounds. Like all seals, leopard seals are naturally inquisitive, but for the most part would rather have nothing at all to do with humans. Birds, especially penguins, top the list of preferred foods, but hard times will send leopard seals to the fish market, and they are not opposed to hunting down and eating other species of seals, some of which are two or three times human size. When they are bothered, most notably when they are being attacked by human hunters for their hides or when the males have formed a harem for breeding, they sneer and open their large mouths, baring their large teeth but remaining remarkably quiet.

Why You Die

Leopard seals lunge and bite with long, sharp teeth that curve inward. They don't chew. They grip with their powerful jaw muscles and shake their heads until something small enough to swallow whole rips off their prey. Not the smallest shred of evidence exists indicating that leopard seals eat human meat. But nonetheless they are most definitely capable of being pressed hard enough to kill.

To Live

Streamlined, with a strong and flexible neck, agile and mighty swift in the water, they are rather awkward when they haul out on land or ice, meaning an average man or woman should be able to outrun an outraged leopard seal.

Moral: The unwise often seal their own doom.

51

SUNK BY SEA LION

There is need for some kind of make-believe
in order to face death unflinchingly.

ERIC HOFFER, 1951

Unlike true seals, sea lions (or eared seals) have external ear flaps, extra-long fore flippers, and rear flippers that rotate. The flippers of sea lions allow them quite a bit of maneuverability out of the ocean. They do a pretty good job of walking on land. Swimming or walking, they are found around the globe, in the Southern and Northern Hemispheres, from the icy sub-Arctic to the warm tropics. Social animals, spending part of their days on rocks or beaches, a hauled-out group may number greater than 1,000. All members of the family Otariidae, they are further divided into six genera, including the California sea lion, the South American sea lion, and the Australian sea lion. They are all large fish-eating carnivores, but none reaches near the size of the Steller sea lion (*Eumetopias jubatus*), whose weight often exceeds a ton and whose length reaches 10 feet. They have big mouths and big teeth, and some of the teeth are pointy and designed for grabbing and holding on tightly to prey. As with true seals, they do not chew—they tear apart and swallow their food. And they are territorial, both in water and on land.

Death by Merciless Mammal

Why You Die

Human–sea lion relationships favor humans. Historically hunted for their meat and their skin, sea lions, especially Steller sea lions, are declining in number. Fishermen also kill them because they are competition. Although well-documented attacks are on record, sea lions rarely harm humans. Your best chance is to crowd one. Coming within 10 feet should do it. They have attacked kayakers, but it's usually during mating season on land that the territorial male will rush over to savagely bite you. If the bite is savage enough, you will bleed to death.

To Live

Give all sea lions the space they deserve. If you accidentally get too close to one, run away at your top speed.

Moral: Allowing personal space is more than a kindness.

52

SLAIN BY SIBERIAN TIGER

Men are convinced of your arguments,
your sincerity, and the seriousness of
your efforts only by your death.

ALBERT CAMUS, 1956

Approximately 40 different wild cats inhabit the earth today, none growing larger than the great Siberian tiger (*Panthera tigris altaica*), which reaches 12 feet in length and 400 to 650 pounds in weight. The greatest of the great tipped the scales at 850 pounds. With a base color of bright reddish orange to white, and bold black stripes, this tiger grows exceptionally long fur to protect it from the intense winters of its range, the vast and frigid Siberian territory. Sometimes covering an area as large as 4,000 square miles, spending most of their time alone and hunting, Siberian tigers have been documented to wander over 600 linear miles in search of food, which, when they are given a choice, will be deer or wild pig. Their immense strength allows them to drag loads that would tax the might of a dozen strong men at once. They need to average about 20 pounds of meat per day to survive, and think nothing of polishing off 100 pounds at one meal. They rarely kill humans, possibly because fewer than 100 of the animals have so far escaped the ravages of *Homo sapiens*.

Death by Merciless Mammal

Why You Die

The Siberian tiger is a stalker, creeping to within 30 to 80 feet before charging an intended victim. Should it happen to be you, you will be grabbed by the neck while the tiger's feet remain firmly planted on the ground. If you survive the initial attack, the tiger will hold on very firmly until you suffocate. Your body will be dragged to a comfortable spot, usually near water, where the cat will feed until satiated. What remains of you will be buried before the tiger takes a break and typically falls asleep. Later you'll be dug up and finished off. Not fun, but definitely interesting.

To Live

Unlike their close kin the Bengal tigers (see "Bested by Bengal Tiger"), Siberian tigers rarely develop a taste for human flesh. Most deaths to humans have occurred during failed attempts to capture one of these cats—so don't do that.

> Moral: You can eat like a pig,
> but don't smell like one.

53

SLUGGED BY SLOTH BEAR

The life of the dead is placed in
the memory of the living.

CICERO, ABOUT 40 BCE

Once thought a relative of the sloth, and thus the name, sloth bears (*Melursus ursinus*) are, well, bears. They have long, shaggy coats of black hair that grows all over, including on their long, floppy ears. The long hair around their heads forms sort of a black mane. Conversely, you can usually see a creamy Y or V on their chest, their muzzle is typically whitish, and their claws are white and exceptionally long. Exceptionally long, too, is the lower lip, allowing them to more easily suck up bugs. Inhabitants of the Indian subcontinent, they are devoted insectivores, eating a great many termites and bees (and their honey) as well as fruit. Averaging 300 pounds or so in weight, they move through a normal day at a sluggish, sloth-like pace, placing their feet heavily and unhurriedly with each step. When aroused, however—which they do get, and often—they are fully capable of running down a human who in turn is running as fast as possible to get away.

Why You Die

Somewhere along the evolutionary timeline, sloth bears decided the best defense is a good offense. Although a sloth bear may run away if you walk up on it, it is far more likely, more likely in fact than most other animals, to stand its ground, roar loudly, and attack. With its long claws, it will strike at your head, especially your face. It will bite your face. In India it is said a week never goes by without a sloth bear attack on a human. Many of those humans who survive are terribly disfigured. And, despite their preference for insects, it is not uncommon for sloth bears to eat a recently killed human.

To Live

Stay indoors at night in sloth bear country since they are nocturnal by nature. Unfortunately, not a lot is known about how best to respond to an attack. Since the bear will probably view you as predator, running away might work. If it catches you, fighting back might work. In either event, good luck.

Moral: Sloth is more than one
of the seven deadly sins.

54

TAMPERED WITH BY TAPIR

> Death is never sweet, not even if it is
> suffered for the highest ideal.
>
> ERICH FROMM, 1941

Inhabitants of jungles and forests in South and Central America and Southeast Asia, the four known species of tapirs (all endangered, all of the genus *Tapirus*) are somewhat piglike in appearance, and whenever possible they spend a lot of time in water. They reach about 7 feet in length and up to 700 pounds in weight, with a short, prehensile snout flexible enough to move in all directions, which allows them to reach the browse they live on (leaves, fruit) that would otherwise be unreachable. Relatives of the rhinoceros, their mouths are filled with chisel-shaped and very strong teeth lodged securely inside very strong jaws.

Thick of skin, and being big, tapirs fall as prey to few predators, and they can run away surprisingly fast, despite the fact that they don't look like they can, disappearing into dense brush or underwater. But cornered or threatened, and especially if they think their young are threatened, they can and will attack.

Why You Die

Tapirs bite. Well-documented stories tell of tapirs delivering severe wounds, even biting off arms. Only on very rare occasions has a tapir been inclined to bite more than once, and the bitten human has bled to death, tapering off slowly. You could therefore be added to a very short list of reasons to die if you are permanently tipped over by a tapir.

To Live
Never threaten a tapir.

Moral: Nosing around can get
you into big trouble.

55

VANQUISHED BY VAMPIRE BAT

> All I know is that I must soon die,
> but what I know least is this very
> death which I cannot escape.
>
> BLAISE PASCAL, 1670

Truly marvelous among the adaptations of nature are the changes in forelimbs that allow a mammal to fly, and no mammal has made this adaptation except the bat. Of the more than 900 species of bats on earth, only 3 are truly blood-sucking vampires, bats that live entirely off blood: the common vampire (*Desmodus rotundus*), the white-winged vampire (*Diaemus youngi*), and the hairy-legged vampire (*Diphylla ecaudata*). They have no regard for the source of the red fluid. Human to toad, it's just food to bats. They find suitable habitat primarily in the tropics and subtropics of the Americas.

Vampire bats home in with their keen sense of smell, with remarkable heat receptors in and below their fatty noses, and with echolocation (in which they emit screams too high-pitched for humans to hear and listen for the echo off whatever they're headed for). With needle-sharp incisors they bite, preferring in humans a small, blood-filled body part such as finger or toe, nose or cheek. Once they create the characteristic V-shaped wounds, they slobber into the opening, their saliva delivering an anticoagulant to keep the blood flowing. Vampire bats don't actually suck, but instead lap up the red

Death by Merciless Mammal

stuff with their tongues. They'll lap for 20 to 30 minutes if you leave them alone.

Why You Die

One bat would not remove enough blood to kill you. In fact, a half dozen probably wouldn't. To be totally honest, nobody knows exactly how many vampire bats would have to feed for how many minutes before you'd reach your expiration date. Nobody has ever been willing to let them feed that long. The immediate danger is far greater from the germs bats may have in their mouths (see "Ravaged by Rabies").

To Live

If a vampire bat bites, swat it, slap it, or grab it and toss it away. Wash the wound aggressively with soap and water for at least 10 minutes, and then find a doctor.

Moral: Bats don't "suck."

> Do not seek death. Death will find you. But seek the road which makes death a fulfillment.
>
> DAG HAMMARSKJÖLD, 1964

All the pinnipeds of the world (seals, sea lions, walruses) are eaters of flesh, but their diets are limited to fish, squid, octopus, shellfish, and occasionally a bird. They have no interest in eating humans, but they can be dangerous, even life threatening to an unwary man or woman. Take the walruses, for instance, creatures that mature at nearly a ton and a half for males and a ton for females.

Walruses (*Odobenus rosmarus rosmarus* in the Atlantic, *O. rosmarus divergens* in the Pacific) of both sexes have flattened, mollusk-crushing teeth except for their two enormously elongated canines, their tusks. They live only in the northern climes of Earth, and they are brightly intelligent with a well-developed fear of humans.

Why You Die

During breeding season or when the mothers have young in their keeping, walruses can develop quarrelsome attitudes and have been known to attack passersby and small boats. When wounded they generally stop at little that holds promise of retaliation. Walruses will throw their huge bulk at you, and if they land as planned, you will be squashed to a shadow

Death by Merciless Mammal

of your former self. Although they don't appear to aim a tusk at you, if a tusk happens to catch you, you'll be ripped from stem to stern.

To Live

They are not exceptionally fast on land, so you should be able to outrun an enraged walrus if you have a decent head start and not too much ice underfoot.

> Moral: A great show of teeth is
> not necessarily a smile.

57

WIPED OUT BY WARTHOG

*Death holds no horrors. It is simply
the ultimate horror of life.*

JEAN GIRAUDOUX, 1933

The world enjoys a plethora of wild pigs: javelinas (peccaries) of the southwestern United States, razorbacks of the southeastern United States, wild boars of Europe. Although not given over totally to vegetarianism, they never hunt large animals, such as humans, for food. They do, however, possess short tempers and a determined willingness to kill when aroused (see "Written Off by Wild Hog"). A peccary hunter in Mexico who was chased up a tree once reported, "They were chewing the tree, and climbing over each other trying to get at me. Each shot laid one out, and each shot seemed to make them more and more furious, as they would rush at the tree, and gnaw the bark and wood, while white flakes of froth fell from their mouths."

African swine of the genus *Phacochoerus* are distinguished by large wart-like protuberances on either side of their remarkably fierce faces and four large, sharp tusks that curve upward from their perpetually sneering lips. Three to four feet long, they are typically reddish gray in color with a bristly black mane and spinal stripe. Poor eyesight is compensated for with a keen sense of smell. They are courageous, ferocious, and really dirty fighters.

Death by Merciless Mammal

Why You Die

When threatened, or even sometimes just approached, warthogs may attack, and usually en masse, thrashing wildly from right to left, up and down, with lunges of their powerful necks, wielding their tusks like a mad drunk with a knife in a city alley. They will rip the tendons out of your legs in order to bring you down to their level. But the ripping has only begun. By the time they're satisfied, you'll cover far more square footage than you used to.

To Live

Give warthogs, especially a clan, plenty of room and no reason to feel threatened. If attacked, run away very fast and/or climb a sturdy tree.

Moral: Stick to pork from the butcher shop.

58

WRITTEN OFF BY WILD HOG

> After all, to the well-organized mind,
> death is but the next great adventure.
>
> J. K. ROWLING, 1991

Once upon a time, all wild hogs (aka wild pigs, feral pigs, feral swine, and some other names) were tame—that is, they were domestic animals that escaped servitude and ran wild, and their descendants not only continue to run amok but also are multiplying. As of right now, they thrive in many countries and 45 of the 50 United States, and the total US population may be as high as eight million. They seem to really like Texas, but they do well in lots of different habitats except where it gets really cold in winter. They can reach over 1,000 pounds in captivity, but 300 pounds in weight seems more like a big one in the wild, and they are hefty up front and sort of smallish toward the back end, with short legs and large canine teeth that sometimes protrude from their mouths. A close relative is the warthog (see "Wiped Out by Warthog"). They are all descended from the wild boar (*Sus scrofa*), who is not tame, and they are all capable of aggressively attacking, especially if one of them feels cornered. Most attacks on humans have been by a solitary hog, but attacks by groups, called sounders, of hogs are well documented. Why they attack is not well studied—sometimes they attack when they are being hunted by humans and sometimes they attack a lone human for unknown reasons.

Why You Die
Injuries to humans are typically to the legs since that's where a wild hog's teeth easily reach. If you fall down, it will go for your abdomen. And that's when you'll really bleed in great spurts, and that's why you'll die.

To Live
Climb a tree—or anything that puts you out of the reach of their teeth. Wild hogs cannot climb. If there's nothing to climb, run away as fast as you can. They don't like to run, and there is a good chance they will lose interest.

Moral: Mean pigs suck.

59

WORRIED BY WOLF

> All that live must die, passing
> through nature to eternity.
>
> WILLIAM SHAKESPEARE, 1600 OR SO

Once wandering over much of the world in tight-knit family groups, wolves now inhabit only remote wilderness areas, generally speaking, and find it more and more difficult to earn a wolfish living. Humans, again generally speaking, fear them and/or don't like them, and often kill them or at least ruin where they like to live. North America provides limited habitat in the western United States and Canada for *Canis lupus*, the gray wolf (also found in Eurasia), and *Canis rupus*, the red wolf—although the red wolf has almost disappeared from the southeastern United States, where it used to be common. The gray wolf (aka timber wolf, western wolf) grows larger than the red, may weigh more than 100 pounds, and may not necessarily be gray but tan, brown, black, even white.

Wolf attacks on humans are rare. If you're interested, your best chance of being the victim of wolves lies outside North America. In the second half of the 20th century, about 200 humans died from wolf bites in southern Asia, but, during the same time period, only 2 humans in the Western Hemisphere suffered that fate.

Why You Die

Wolves hunt as they live, in packs, and a really hungry pack—"starving" might be a better descriptor—will surround you, taking turns dashing in for a nip. Eventually you'll fall to the ground, where they will concentrate on your head and neck. This part can hurt a lot, but it won't last long. Jaws powerful enough to break large bones will break yours, dividing you up, mouthful by bloody mouthful, among the pack until you are gone.

To Live

Fight back! Wolves are accustomed to dinner trying to escape but not dinner hitting them on their noses with sticks and rocks.

Moral: "Wolfing down food" has more than one meaning.

DEATH BY BODACIOUS BIRD

All members of the class Aves have feathers covering warm-blooded bodies, lightweight yet strong skeletons, and beaks that open on toothless mouths, and the females lay hard-shelled eggs. There are about 10,000 species spread all around the world. They are often very pretty, and they often sing very pretty songs. Almost all of them can fly, almost all of them are harmless, and almost everybody already knows this stuff about birds. But there are exceptions: large angry birds that can kill humans.

60

CASTRATED BY CASSOWARY

Neither the sun nor death can
be looked at steadily.

FRANÇOIS DE LA ROCHEFOUCAULD, 1665

One of the few types of birds, perhaps even the only one, to go out of its way to attack humans, the cassowary (comprising three species in genus *Casaurius*), a distant relative of the ostrich and emu, lives only in Australia, New Guinea, and adjacent islands. It often stands more than 6 feet tall and tends to top everybody's list of the world's most dangerous birds. Generally dark greenish in color, loose and coarse, its plumage hangs down like thick hair that has lost its interest in life. The head and neck are brightly colored, usually blue with other tints visible, and on top of the head sits a helmet-like structure of unknown use. With wings too small for flight, cassowaries may reach 130 pounds in weight at maturity and run speedily across the ground on powerful legs that end in feet with a long, straight, strong, sharp claw on the three toes. The claw on each of the two innermost toes can grow up to 5 inches long. Since they choose one mate and the two stick together, when you see a lone cassowary it probably isn't—the other one is lurking nearby. Remarkably dumb with a reputation for "flying" completely into hysterics, quarrelsome and combative in nature, cassowaries, when surprised in the bush, may charge regardless of what disturbed them.

Why You Die

Before slamming into you, at a precisely timed moment, they'll leap into the air and slash out and down with their knifelike claws. Any part of you in the path of the claws will be ripped open the way you tear into a recalcitrant bag of corn chips. The attack may be formidable and prolonged, depending on how resistant you are, sometimes ending with you still and lifeless.

To Live

If you are suddenly overcome with a deep desire to see tomorrow, forget outrunning a cassowary. Try throwing yourself to the ground, curling up, covering everything vital with your arms, and hoping for the best.

Moral: Birds of a feather freak out together.

61 EDGED OUT BY EAGLE

> Life is pleasant. Death is peaceful. It's
> the transition that's troublesome.
>
> ISAAC ASIMOV, MIGHT HAVE BEEN 1960

"Eagle" ranks among commonly heard names, even outside of Philadelphia, and when the subject is the family Accipitridae (the eagles that are birds), there are at least 60 species worldwide. Only 2 of the 60 are native to North America, the bald eagle and the golden eagle. The majority of them are either African or Eurasian, but nine species live in this hemisphere, well south of the US border, and three are Australian. They are all birds of prey with large wings that they tuck in for stunningly fast dives. The bald eagle, for instance, has been clocked at 99 miles per hour during a headfirst plummet toward earth. Their size, their speed, their beaks powered by muscles that allow them to carnivorously rip meat apart, and their talons that can clamp down with literally bone-crushing strength make the eagle a potentially dangerous-to-humans bird. The death of an eagle's prey begins when the powerful talons sink in. Anything surviving the tremendous squeeze gets a spine-ripping attack by the beak.

Why You Die

And now for a moment of truth: No human deaths have been attributed to eagles. But possibilities exist. Something weighing between 12 and 15 pounds, traveling at 99 miles per hour, and slamming into the side of your head would probably end your life. Witnesses have filmed eagles pulling much larger animals off of cliffs, watching them fall, and dropping down to feast. An eagle would not eat you, but one could unbalance you on a precipitous edge. And then, given a really disastrous-for-you situation, an eagle could theoretically rip out your throat.

To Live
Do nothing to upset an eagle.

Moral: Live and let live.

62

OBLITERATED BY OSTRICH

Even at our birth, death does but stand aside
a little. And every day he looks towards us
and muses somewhat to himself whether
that day or the next he will draw nigh.

ROBERT BOLT, 1962

Not far removed from reptiles, birds are hardly more than warm-blooded lizards with a few other differences such as feathers instead of scales. Birds are creatures of very small brains, which gave rise to the expression "bird-brained," which means, in short, not very smart. Most animals substantially smaller than you will back off when you fight back, but not necessarily birds. Even some tiny birds will fly at you again and again if they put their tiny minds to it. This is rarely a problem—unless the bird is not tiny.

The ostrich, a great flightless bird of Africa, is the largest bird on earth. This black-and-white bird runs fast and reaches heights of nearly 8 feet and weights of around 300 pounds. Since ostriches are valued for their feathers and the taste of their meat, ostrich farms are springing up around the world, including in the United States. And the ostrich is one of the few birds that will attack a human just because the bird is having a bad day. When mating season rolls around, the male ostrich, the cock, is considered by some experts to be among the most volatile and dangerous animals on the surface of the planet.

Why You Die

Ostriches give a terrifically powerful kick with either of their piston-like legs, legs of which the lower half is virtually solid bone ending in razor-keen claws on two toes. Given the right mood and a chance, they'll kick out and down, ripping the guts from your abdomen and stringing them along the ground as they step in for another kick.

139

To Live

Interesting to note is the fact that ostriches, even the most hysterical cocks, will not kick at or even step on a human lying flat on the ground—although they might peck at you for a bit.

Moral: There's much to be said for a low profile.

63

WRESTLED DOWN BY RHEA

Death is a delightful hiding place for weary men.
HERODOTUS, SOMEWHERE NEAR 400 BCE

There are two of them, if you are counting species: the greater rhea (*Rhea americana*) and the lesser rhea (*Rhea pennata*). When they run—which they can do at 40 miles per hour—their wings open and close as if they wish they could take off, but they cannot. As with ostriches, rheas are flightless. They look like ostriches, too, with long necks and long legs, but they are smaller than ostriches with heads rising, in an adult greater rhea, about 5.5 feet off the ground and with bodies weighing in at most around 90 pounds. Natives of South America, they flutter their grayish-brown, tattered-looking plumage in open grasslands from Brazil and Peru down through Bolivia and Argentina. Unexpectedly, a mated pair or two escaped in Germany in the 1990s, and a flock of more than 100 thrives there. You will see them nowhere else, except in captivity.

If you get a peek at a rhea's feet, you will see only three toes. They do not have a rear toe like most birds do. At the end of each toe is a stout toenail. Male rheas gather the eggs of several females and sit on them until they hatch. That's when a rhea gets testy and aggressive, attacking anything that comes near the nest, even female rheas, and that's when their powerful legs and long toes can be dangerous.

Death by Bodacious Bird

Why You Die

As ostriches do (see "Obliterated by Ostrich"), an outraged rhea kicks out and down with enough strength to tear open your abdomen and spill your insides to the outside. Fortunately, rheas are generally timid, preferring running away to standing and fighting. But why tempt one?

To Live

You can't outrun a rhea, but a hurried retreat by you will likely discourage one. If the bird fails to be discouraged, drop to the ground, facedown, and cover your head with your arms.

Moral: A bird in hand is sometimes a really bad idea.

DEATH BY AQUATIC ACCIDENT

Eventually you need to come up for air, and denizens of the deep (or shallow) do not, excepting a few creatures such as whales, who can hold their breath far, far longer than you can. Not being able to get to air definitely tops the list of reasons for humans to die in water. But there are more. Waterborne reasons to perish include animals with big teeth and other body parts that may cause you to bleed too much and animals that harbor deadly poisons.

64

BAGGED BY BARRACUDA

> The whole life of instinct serves the
> one end of bringing about death.
>
> SIGMUND FREUD, 1920

Tropical and subtropical seas worldwide provide a home for
22 species of swift, meat-eating fish, family Sphyraenidae, collectively known as barracudas, but with few exceptions they
bother humans very little. One exception is the great barracuda, *Sphyraena barracuda*, which grows to nearly 6 feet in
length, has a huge mouth filled with two sets of noticeably
sharp teeth, and has been known to attack and kill humans.
Inquisitive by nature and sight oriented, barracudas are built
for incredible speed, and they use speed to suddenly flash out
of "nowhere" to snag their prey. They bite humans less often

than sharks do, but hitting so fast and so hard, a 5-foot-long specimen could remove enough tissue in one chomp to end your life.

Why You Die

Deeply and raggedly lacerated, you bleed to death before you can get on board or to shore in time to staunch the flow.

To Live

Barracudas couldn't care less about whether you taste good. Although ultimately unpredictable, they are stimulated to attack for much the same reasons that sharks bite humans: (1) The water is murky and the barracuda can't tell if you're a regular food source or something new, larger than its normal lunch, and possibly unappealing. (2) You are wearing a flashy swimsuit or carrying some sort of shiny paraphernalia that appears to the barracuda to be the belly of another fish—in other words, a meal. (3) You are an angler or a spearfisher toting a string of bleeding fish, an obvious attraction. (4) You have been messing around with the barracuda, maybe trying to catch it or maybe just swimming in too close for its comfort. And one more thing: Big, solitary barracudas are more likely to attack than those traveling in schools. So to avoid getting bitten, avoid the foregoing situations.

Moral: When school lets out,
it's time to go home.

65

BULLIED BY BULL SHARK

> You may complete as many generations as you please during your life; none the less will that everlasting death await you.
>
> LUCRETIUS, FIRST CENTURY BCE

Humans who fish for fun and profit haul an estimated and astounding 100 million sharks over their gunwales every year. These sharks die, often after being dumped live back into the ocean with their dorsal fins cut off. No wonder some sharks, notably the bull shark (*Carcharhinus leucas*), are apt to take the opportunity now and then to bully a human. Bull sharks, in fact, are one of the three shark species most likely to feed on a human (see "Gobbled by Great White Shark" and "Torn Apart by Tiger Shark").

Bull sharks may rip into more humans than any other species, and they are considered by many experts to be the most dangerous man-eaters in tropical seas. One reason bull sharks rate high on the danger list is an unusual habit they have: They swim regularly up freshwater rivers, including the Amazon (South America), Bombay (Asia), Brisbane (Australia), Congo (Africa), and lower Mississippi (North America). Brown, black, or gray in color, growing to 11 feet in length, bull sharks can weigh well over 400 pounds. Among the least picky about their food of all sharks, bulls are wonderfully opportunistic, eating whatever whenever they have a chance, but feeding primarily at dawn and dusk. Beady of eye and blunt of nose, these sharks have a very large mouth filled with very large serrated teeth.

Why You Die

Bull sharks have a tendency to head-butt food before biting, perhaps to make sure the intended meal is edible. If you pass the initial inspection, they'll raise their snout to perfectly line up their gaping jaws for a bite that will remove a very large portion of you. You can bleed to death rather quickly.

To Live

Here are five things you do not want to do in water potentially bull shark infested: (1) Swim with the sharks. (2) Bleed while swimming with the sharks. (3) Swim when the water is murky. (4) Swim alone. (5) Swim at night.

Moral: Nobody likes a bully.

Death by Aquatic Accident

66

CANNED BY CANDIRU

> Death in itself is nothing; but we fear to be
> we know not what, we know not where.

JOHN DRYDEN, 1682

The size of a small toothpick, an inch or so long, the candiru is a translucent, almost invisible catfish, an inhabitant of Amazonian waters, a parasite (which is most unusual among fish). The candiru sucks blood, most often by attaching itself to the gills of larger fish, drinking until it is satiated, and dropping off to rest on the bottom until it gets hungry again. To the utter devastation of a few humans, mentally and sometimes physically, candirus have a serious problem distinguishing between the smell of blood-rich fish gills and the smell of human urine. They swim up into the urethra of peeing people, or perhaps into other urogenital openings. They expand their spike-like gills, and that holds them in place in fish gills while they feed; then they swim forward and out. In a human urethra, of course, there isn't an out to swim. They are very, very securely stuck inside.

Why You Die

This minuscule catfish, sometimes called the urethra fish in English (*candiru* is Portuguese), will not live long inside you. After it dies you will become progressively septicemic, dying in misery from blood poisoning.

To Live

In Amazonian males, early methods of treatment included whacking off, in a most literal sense, the penis. This may help explain the low population growth rate in some areas of Amazonia. Large doses of citric acid have now been proven to soften the spike-like gills and often encourage the release and resulting expulsion of the candiru. Despite tales to the contrary, they cannot swim up a stream of urine. You have to be peeing while you're at least partially submerged—so don't do that.

> **Moral:** The Amazon basin may be an excellent opportunity for someone who sells snug-fitting swimsuits.

67

CEASED BY CIGUATERA

In the depth of the anxiety of having to die
is the anxiety of being eternally forgotten.

PAUL TILLICH, 1963

More commonly diagnosed than any other fish-related illness, ciguatera poisoning follows ingestion by humans of several types of tropical and subtropical reef fish in the Pacific and Caribbean, especially but not only snapper, grouper, kingfish, amberjack, barracuda, dolphin (the fish one), wrasse, sturgeon fish, goatfish, and parrot fish.

Tiny dinoflagellate marine algae called *Gambierdiscus toxicus*, when eaten by herbivorous reef fish, produce toxins that concentrate in the guts of the fish. Among those toxins are ciguatoxin and ciguaterin. When humans eat these vegetarian fish, or the carnivorous fish that have eaten the vegetarians, poisoning occurs. Ciguatera toxins give the fish no unusual odor, taste, or color, and they are resistant to freezing, cooking, drying, and smoking. What happens in the sea to produce the dinoflagellates is not known. It's a big problem for fish eaters who want to live in the South Pacific, Japan, the Bahamas, Hawaii, Puerto Rico, or Florida, and ciguatera poisoning has been diagnosed at least two dozen times in Baja California.

Why You Die

Within 24 hours of ingesting toxic fish, you'll usually complain of gastrointestinal symptoms: nausea, vomiting, abdominal pain, and diarrhea. In mild poisonings these symptoms resolve quickly, but they may last for as long as a week. Neurologic symptoms include paresthesia (strange skin sensations), vertigo, ataxia (loss of coordination), myalgia (muscle pain), weakness, headache, cold/hot sensory reversal, joint pain, and itching. Weirdest is an occasional complaint of feeling like your teeth are loose. These symptoms, too, spontaneously resolve, but may reoccur from time to time over the next few years. Cardiovascular symptoms occur only in patients who have been severely poisoned and may include tachycardia (fast heart rate), bradycardia (slow heart rate), and hypotension (low blood pressure). Sometimes symptoms are worse on a second exposure to the toxins. Although it is rare, the cardiovascular challenges have permanently done in a few humans.

To Live

Although ciguatera poisoning has no specific antidote, supportive care means almost everyone will go on living.

> Moral: There's something more
> than fishy about some fish.

68

CAPTURED BY GIANT CLAM

Every death, even the cruelest, drowns in
the total indifference of Nature; Nature
herself would watch unmoved if we
destroyed the entire human race.

PETER WEISS, 1964

Pearl divers of the Indo-Pacific region, off many South Pacific
island groups and off the coast of East Africa, insist that the
giant clam (*Tridacna gigas*), the world's largest mollusk, is a

threat to life. Without their shells their soft body parts may weigh in at 20 pounds or more, a hefty meal for the mollusk eater but hardly a menace. The shell, however, of this humongous bivalve (sometimes called the killer clam or man-eating clam) may exceed 4 feet in length and reach almost 500 pounds in weight. The strength of the adductor muscles required to shut the shell, as you can imagine, is immense.

The *US Navy Diving Manual* rates the giant clam a 2-plus (out of a possible high mark of 4-plus) on the danger scale and says, "Traps arms and legs between shells." With serrated edges, the two halves of the shell fit together like the jaws of a mighty bear trap and as tightly as pearl buyers grip their money.

Why You Die

On behalf of giant clams, let it be known that they do not eat humans. A vast weight of evidence indicates that these mollusks are innocent undersea bystanders prompted by nothing other than a tickle to their "trapdoor." Victims simply freak out and struggle until they drown.

To Live

The *US Navy Diving Manual* gives specific instructions about cutting the clam's adductor muscles in order to release your trapped body part.

Moral: Never look a gift pearl-bearer in the eye.

Death by Aquatic Accident

69

CONKED BY CONE SHELL

I have seen the eternal Footman
hold my coat, and snicker.

T. S. ELIOT, 1915

Among the most delicate and beautiful of color of any sea-shells are cone shells. Between 400 and 500 species (genus *Conus*) exist, and they are all equipped with a highly developed apparatus for envenomation. Found in tropical and subtropical seas, cone shells live on rocks and coral and sometimes are seen crawling along sandy bottoms. Generally shy and retiring, the animals inside cone shells hide when approached. But they strike out violently when the shell is handled.

Once the cone shell is in your hand, a snout shoots out of the shell's opening, a fleshy snout of remarkable length. The snout contains quite a few rigid, hollow tools called radula teeth that will quickly penetrate your skin, even through gloves. The wound looks like a scrape. Each harpoon-like tooth has its own separate venom supply that enters your body. On the low end of "bad," some cone shells' venom provides pain like the worst bee sting you can imagine, but on the upper end, death can occur in less than four hours. With a 20 percent mortality rate, cone shells rank statistically higher than cobras and rattlesnakes as death-dealing devices.

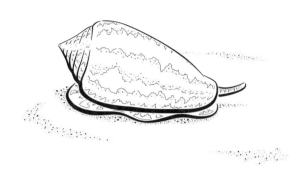

Why You Die

Besides pain, you should feel tingling and numbness, especially in your lips and mouth, followed shortly by a creeping paralysis in your arms and legs. Be prepared for some dizziness and vomiting. As the paralysis spreads to your diaphragm, you'll find it more and more difficult to first talk and then breathe. If you got scraped by one of the less venomous species, these problems will pass. If you handled one of the more venomous species, you will soon lose consciousness and expire when your breathing stops.

To Live

Apply a pad that covers the site of the sting and a couple of inches above and below the site. Wrap an elastic bandage around the pad, pressing it firmly in place but not tight enough to cut off circulation—and find a doctor.

Moral: Keep your hands to yourself.

70

CRACKED BY CRAB

Grieve not; though the journey of life be
bitter, and the end unseen, there is no
road which does not lead to an end.

HAFIZ, 14TH CENTURY CE

Humans have regularly hunted crabs for food ever since that distant day when someone discovered they tasted good. On the shores and islands of the South Pacific, the Indian Ocean, and the adjacent seas lives a much-sought-after crustacean, *Birgus latro*, the robber crab or coconut crab. It grows to over a foot in length and is culinarily just fine when boiled and cracked open, and the meat picked out and dipped in warm butter. Crabs have always had a chance to return the compliment when a dead human ended up in their domain, although they simply tear a corpse apart and eat it disgustingly soggy and raw. Coconut crabs get some revenge by commonly carrying a toxin that can make humans sick. Occasionally—if truth be told, very rarely—*Birgus* does more.

These creatures are called coconut crabs for a remarkable reason: They scuttle sideways from the sea to climb palms and pinch off coconuts, causing them to fall to the sand. Then they descend to tear the coconuts apart. Then they eat the good stuff inside each coconut. They, in other words, have very powerful pincers.

Why You Die

One account from 1951, this on an island in the Red Sea, reports that shipwrecked Muslim sailors were dozing weakly on the beach. Coconut crabs emerged silently from their salty home to crack open the skulls (and kill) 26 humans before the survivors awoke and retaliated. Perhaps the crabs mistook the hairy human heads for coconuts. Perhaps they, at last, had an opportunity for true revenge.

To Live

Do not nap on the beach in coconut crab country.

Moral: Bald is beautiful.

71 | EXTERMINATED BY ELECTRIC EEL

Rich man and poor move side by
side toward the limit of death.

PINDAR, FIFTH CENTURY BCE

Though decidedly eel-like in appearance, electric eels (*Electrophorus electricus*), growing up to 10 feet in length and 90 pounds in weight, are not true eels but fish of shallow freshwater in Brazil, Colombia, Peru, and perhaps surrounding countries. The electric eel is not even a normal fish, as it breathes air and will drown if held underwater for 15 minutes or so, something you most assuredly do not want to do to one. All its vital organs are found a short distance behind its head and after that is a long stretch of electricity-producing tissue. Discharges of electricity from eels have been measured at 650 volts, and far less can end your life.

These creatures surround themselves with an electric field with which they navigate and sense their prey, a process that becomes more and more important to eels as they mature and lose what little eyesight they possess. They stun their prey and then consume the fishy meal while it's still alive. Eels have no interest in dead fish. They cannot control their voltage, but they can control the number of pulses of electricity they discharge. Pulses start from a point about one-fifth of the way tail-ward from the head and run the length of the body to end at the tail.

Why You Die

Fatal contact with an electric eel results when your heart is stopped by the charge, but you can be knocked unconscious more than 20 feet away and drown (see "Suffocated by Submersion") while you're in the water with one.

To Live

While in Brazil, Colombia, and Peru, limit your swimming to the pool at the hotel. If you fail to follow this advice, CPR might work.

Moral: Some people get more of a charge out of life than they ever expected.

> What good can come from meeting
> death with tears? . . . If a man is sorry
> for himself, he doubles death.
>
> EURIPIDES, 414 BCE

Who knows what may lurk in the dark of the deeps? At least 300 species of sharks have been identified, ranging in size at maturity from 6 inches to almost 50 feet (see "Bullied by Bull Shark" and "Torn Apart by Tiger Shark"). But teeth have been found—the same teeth that grow in the mouths of great white sharks—that measured 5 inches long. Such teeth fell from the mouth of a white shark that had grown to 100 feet in length. No shark that size has ever been recorded, but the teeth were not fossils!

Dark blue, gray, gray-green, even brown on top, great white sharks (*Carcharodon carcharias*) are only white on the bottom half. With no bones, just cartilage, and virtually no brain, white sharks are huge stretches of death-dealing muscle, the evolutionary pinnacle of a waterborne killing machine. At maximum weights that approach two tons, these sharks tend to kill and swallow large things: seals and sea lions, salmon, tuna, dolphins, great turtles, and now and then a human. Totally fearless, great whites are the only sharks, the only fish, that will lift their eyes above the water to spot prey. To a great white shark, a human kicking along the surface of the ocean, especially on a surfboard, is just another tasty morsel, something that looks sort of like some of their regular food. They seem to develop a taste for, or at least do not mind the taste of, humans (see the movie *Jaws*).

Why You Die

Their attacks are sudden, swift, and terrifying: one huge bite from a huge mouth full of huge teeth. Then they back off and wait until their food bleeds to death. Sharks in general detest a struggle, and they are magnificently patient. Take all the time you want to bleed to death.

To Live

If you can get out of the water alive, apply direct pressure to your wound until the bleeding stops. If a part of you is missing, you may require a tourniquet on what's left of you to stop the bleeding. After that find a doctor.

> Moral: Sometimes tasting good
> means more than good taste.

73

HAMMERED BY HAMMERHEAD

A man's dying is more the
survivors' affair than his own.

THOMAS MANN, 1924

Of all the shark species on earth (see "Gobbled by Great
White Shark"), only 21 species have been well documented
to have killed humans. Of those 21, the sharks represented
in this book—great white, tiger, bull, and hammerhead—are
the ones most likely to kill a human. None is more regularly
unpredictable than the hammerhead sharks (genus *Sphyrna*),
of which there are nine species, weird-looking fish with eyes

at either end of hammer-shaped heads. The hammer shape, called a cephalofoil, may help them glide through the water, but no one knows for sure. Three species of hammerheads—great, scalloped, and smooth—are among the 21 known killers of *Homo sapiens*, but it doesn't happen very often, and some experts declare hammerheads do not belong among the Big Four. Despite the seemingly awkward placement of their jaws beneath the "hammer," and despite the fact that their mouths and teeth are small for a shark, hammerheads are precise killers of their natural food sources.

Like most sharks, hammerheads have gill slits but no way to flap their gills, so they must stay in motion to breathe, forcing oxygen-rich water across their gills, all their lives. This may explain in part their tendency to be irritable. Hammerheads, especially the great hammerhead, which can reach a length of around 20 feet and a weight of nearly 1,000 pounds, can carry a load of irritability. But the fear all sharks induce in humans is not reflected in their kill rate, their attacks being fatal about 30 times a year worldwide.

Why You Die

A hammerhead that decides to bite will swim in quickly, raising its head at the final moment to take out a chunk of flesh. For a shark it won't be a tremendously huge chunk, but you might bleed to death before you reach safety—unless it comes back for another bite, in which case you will likely bleed to death.

To Live

If you are confronted by a hammerhead, or any shark, and you suddenly discover you want to live, face the shark and stay as calm as possible. If the shark approaches close enough, try kicking, punching, and gouging its eyes, none of which will hurt the shark in the least but some of which might discourage it. If you are alone, swimming away as fast as you can is utterly useless.

> Moral: When in shark-infested waters, always swim with someone who swims a lot slower than you.

74

JUMPED BY JELLYFISH

Do not rejoice over anyone's death;
remember that we all must die.

ECCLESIASTICUS 8:7

Not really a fish, so you might see the "fish" part of the name disappear soon, jellyfish belong to the phylum Coelenterata, the coelenterates, which includes sea anemones, corals, and hydroids (see "Mangled by Man-of-War"). From almost microscopic species to the giant lion's mane jellyfish (*Cyanea capillata*), with a body over 7 feet in diameter and tentacles dangling down more than 100 feet, true jellyfish drift on the sea of life in all the oceans of earth. Some cause humans no harm at all. Some cause humans mild pain, and some cause screaming pain. A few cause an agonizing death.

Jellyfish work this way: Their tentacles are covered in specialized stinging organelles called nematocysts that are contained in specialized cells called cnidoblasts. Each cnidoblast has a cnidocil, a "trigger," that activates the cell when something, such as a human, touches it. A "trapdoor" called an operculum flies open and a spring-loaded, microscopic, barbed venom sac plunges into, let's say, an arm. One swipe of the arm through the tentacles of a jellyfish can stimulate thousands to hundreds of thousands of nematocysts to fire out their venomous daggers. No jellyfish attack humans.

Death by Aquatic Accident

They just automatically sting everything they bump into, hoping it will turn out to be food.

Why You Die

If you're swimming, you're likely to panic and drown (see "Suffocated by Submersion"). But the box jellyfish (*Chironex fleckeri*), sometimes mistakenly called a sea wasp (which is another dangerous jellyfish, *Carybdea marsupialis*), is common from the Philippines to Australia and carries one of the world's deadliest venoms, often killing in less than 10 minutes, sometimes in as little as 30 seconds! If you have time after being stung, you'll notice profound muscle spasms and muscular and respiratory paralysis. You won't notice, but your blood pressure will drop. Suddenly your heart will stop, and it's the deep six for you.

To Live

Get out of the water. Rinse your pain-rich skin with seawater. Do not rub it or apply ice. Rinse a second time with vinegar, or alcohol if that's what you have. Scrape off the attached tentacles, if any, but not with your bare hand. Shave the affected skin with a razor or knife, or anything with an edge. If you swam into a box jellyfish, you should find the antivenin ASAP.

Moral: Just because something is smaller than you doesn't mean you should push it around.

75

KAYOED BY KILLER WHALE

Pity is for the living, envy is for the dead.

MARK TWAIN, 1897

Communal creatures, killer whales (*Orcinus orca*) live in tight-knit herds, also called pods, and have IQs that equal or surpass those of the great apes. Ranging from the Arctic to the Antarctic, largest of the dolphins, warm-blooded and air-breathing, black with attractive smears of white, killer whales grow to over 30 feet in length and undoubtedly deserve their name: They feed regularly on other warm-blooded animals, with seals, penguins, porpoises, and smaller dolphins being by far their favorite foods. Inside their Herculean jaws are conical teeth up to 2 inches across at the base. Speedy of fin, they can swim down any of their chosen food sources. When driven by hunger, they will rise 6 to 8 feet out of the water to spot a meal on a beach or ice floe and throw themselves well up onto land or ice to reach the intended prey. They have been watched repeatedly battering floes in attempts to dislodge seals. Other whales, often substantially larger than killer whales, have been known to launch themselves onto land (where they suffocate, unable to expand their lungs due to their massive body weight) in order to escape the onslaught of a pod of starving orcas.

From centuries of human observation of these mighty animals, a most astounding fact emerges: Not once has

Death by Aquatic Accident

a killer whale ever been proven to kill a human in the wild wet outdoors. Incidents have occurred in which killer whales appeared to attack a human, such as by flopping up onto ice where a human was standing. But these cases are almost undoubtedly examples of mistaken identity. The whales thought they were going for a seal.

Why You Die
It is theoretically possible to be killed if you dive into a pod of hungry killer whales after smearing seal blubber all over yourself. That would definitely put you in the record books.

To Live
Enjoy the wonder of whales from a respectable distance.

> Moral: A whale of a good time is
> more an attitude than an event.

76

MANGLED BY MAN-OF-WAR

Death has but one terror, that
it has no tomorrow.

ERIC HOFFER, 1954

Not a true jellyfish (see "Jumped by Jellyfish"), the Portuguese man-of-war (*Physalia physalia*), or bluebottle, is a hydroid, a colony of specialized animals living together in a highly cooperative state in which different jobs are performed for the benefit of the whole, sort of a sticky glob of Leninist Russia. The blue "bottle" or "balloon," named for a Portuguese sailing ship, is a single overgrown animal filled with air. The tentacles are another type of animal, the stomachs another type, and the reproductive organs still another type. With no organs for elimination, the man-of-war's waste products come back up and out its feeding orifices. The colony has no heart, no brain, and no rectum—just a tummy that can have babies and poops out its mouth. Though the man-of-war is deceptively small on the surface, its tentacles hang down as far as 165 feet below its blue "sail." Blown literally by the winds and currents of fate, the man-of-war may show up anywhere in warm ocean water but appears most often in the mid-Atlantic and the Sargasso Sea, most often in large groups that may include thousands.

Why You Die

Swim into one of these colonies, and you'll experience instant and agonizing pain. Raised welts where the tentacles struck will rise up to red heights. You may feel like a whale has beached on your chest, making it difficult to breathe. Pain may wash through your abdomen and lower back, with muscle cramps extending down your legs and arms. As the venom is nonlethal, the cause of death is most often panic and drowning.

To Live

Try to relax, and get out of the water. Immediately rinse your skin with seawater, not freshwater. Apply soaks of vinegar or isopropyl alcohol. Remove the tentacles still attached to you, but not with your bare hands. Then apply cold to ease the pain.

Moral: Socialism isn't for everyone.

77

MINCED BY MARLIN

Our fear of death is like our fear
that summer will be short . . .

RALPH WALDO EMERSON, 1855

About 10 species of marlin have been named, the "about" resulting from of lack of agreement among taxonomists—who, it appears, are sort of like politicians sitting on opposite sides of the aisle with little (or no) hope of ever coming to an agreement. They, the marlin, are all members of the fish family Istiophoridae. To gain membership in this family you need, among other requirements, an elongated body, a dorsal fin (the one on top) that extends in a crest-like fashion, and—here's the important part—a long and extremely rigid and pointy bill. The bill on average, from eyeball to tip, constitutes approximately 20 percent of a marlin's length, and they use it to stun and kill food sources. Marlins weighing in at 200 pounds have gained enough speed to ram their bills entirely through a 5-inch-thick wooden plank—even though they can't eat a wooden plank. Atlantic blues (*Makaira nigricans*), the biggest marlins, are well documented to exceed 16 feet in elongated body and 1,800 pounds in weight. Despite the name, you can find them in the Pacific and the Indian as well as the Atlantic Ocean. Add their size to the fact that marlins are a prized catch for sport fisherfolk, and you have a setup for fatal encounters.

Death by Aquatic Accident

Why You Die

Powerful swimmers, marlins, when hooked, throw themselves to prodigious heights out of the water and phenomenal distances over the water. More than once these heights and distances have ended with the rigid bill completely through what had only recently been a very excited human being.

To Live

Cast your bait out exclusively for bass and crappies or wear a Kevlar vest when going after marlin. On second thought, wear two Kevlar vests.

Moral: Sometimes it is very important to *not* get the point.

78

OUTWITTED BY OCTOPUS

The end of all is death and man's life passeth away suddenly as a shadow.

THOMAS Á KEMPIS, 1426

With a bulbous, bag-shaped body (called a mantle) and eight arms supplied with two rows of suckers to hold their prey, octopi live worldwide, preferring the warmer tropical and temperate seas. Octopi are mollusks, relatives of squids (see "Squished by Squid"), cuttlefish, and nautiluses, and they hunt by stealth, sneaking up on prey, grabbing crabs, crayfish, and shellfish with their sticky arms, and biting with a beak that hides in the heart of the encircling appendages. Octopi stun their victims with a nerve poison and hang out until the squirming prey squirms no more. Without a means to inject their poison, they are relegated to biting and spitting the poison into the wound. Almost all octopi have venom harmless to humans. Although on rare occasions an unusual octopus, probably a mentally challenged individual, has been known to leap out of the sea and grab a wading man or woman, death via that means has not occurred, at least not a well-documented death.

But don't relax: The colorful and diminutive blue-ringed octopus (genus *Hapalochlaena*) ranks among the deadliest denizens of the deep. Look for blue-ringed octopi off the coasts of eastern and northern Australia, Indonesia, and the

Death by Aquatic Accident

Philippines and up to southern Japan. Blue rings circle their arms and blue crescents highlight their purplish-brown to yellowish bodies. Some blue-ringed octopi are no bigger than a golf ball, and one 10 inches long would be a giant among its peers. When irritated or excited, the rings glow an iridescent peacock blue, which typically happens when an unknowing human picks up one of the little fellows.

Why You Die

The bite is seldom felt, the spit never seen. You may notice a small trickle of blood from the bite site. Within five minutes, maybe a bit more, you'll feel dry in the mouth and have difficulty swallowing as the toxin attacks your nervous system.

You will become rapidly and violently ill—vomiting, losing muscular control, and collapsing on the beach. Your ability to breathe will become paralyzed, and you'll turn a shade of blue far less appealing than the blue of your killer. You'll pass out before you die. The poison is extremely deadly, sometimes causing the bitten human to expire in a brief 90 minutes.

To Live

Wrap the bitten extremity fully in an elastic bandage, and head directly for a hospital. There is no known antidote for the venom, but if you stop breathing and someone performs rescue breathing, your life may be extended. If you make it 24 hours, you'll probably survive.

> Moral: Never embrace anything
> with more arms than you.

79

PARTAKEN OF BY PIRANHA

We must needs die, and are as water spilt on the ground, which cannot be gathered up again.

2 SAMUEL 14:14

Perhaps as many as 30 species of piranhas live in the rivers and lakes of South America, and maybe 20 of those species in the waters of the extensive Amazon basin, but only 4 or 5 of them have ever been known to partake of a human being. Of piranhas, Theodore Roosevelt wrote: "They are the most ferocious fish in the world." Considered by many experts to be the most dangerous piranha, though not the largest, *Serrasalmus nattereri* (the red-bellied piranha) grows to about 11 inches and travels in immense schools. The mouths of all piranhas are not that immense, but they are filled with needle-sharp teeth and they bite with powerful jaws. Relatively irritable when hungry, piranhas will devour each other if kept enclosed for too long without food. When shipped, which sometimes happens, piranhas require one container per fish since that's all you'll end up with anyway.

Why You Die

When blood spills in piranha-infested water, the fish are driven into a veritable feeding frenzy that has reduced many fairly large mammals, including humans, into a pile of bones in remarkably short order, perhaps, say some unsubstantiated reports, less than two minutes.

To Live

To decrease your chances of becoming piranha food, do not swim in murky waters (doing so tricks the fish into thinking you're a normal part of their diet), do not thrash wildly about to imitate something in trouble, and do not bleed.

Moral: Don't feed the fish.

80

POISONED BY PUFFER FISH

For the dead there are no more toils.

SOPHOCLES, AROUND 413 BCE

Of the 120 or so species of puffer fish (family Tetraondontidae), some may grow as long as 3 feet and as heavy as 30 pounds. They mostly prefer the warmth of tropical and subtropical ocean water. When threatened they are unique in that they suck water, or air if water isn't available, into an internal bladder, "puffing" themselves up to two or three times normal size—a deterrent to predators, the puffer fish hopes. Even if eaten by predators, puffer fish get revenge since they contain a highly toxic chemical called tetrodotoxin. Tetrodotoxin is a poison about 1,200 times more dangerous than cyanide and one of the most potent poisons found in nature. If the puffer fish benefits from being poisonous, other than getting revenge after death, it is not understood why.

In Japan, puffer fish—also called blowfish, globefish, and swellfish—precisely prepared, is considered a great delicacy. The Japanese call the dish *fugu*. But improper preparation may give *you* a case of tetrodotoxin poisoning. If your chef toils properly, no organ of the fish touches the soon-to-be-eaten flesh. Death to humans occurs in approximately 60 percent of all cases of puffer fish poisoning, a regular occurrence in less-than-four-star Japanese restaurants.

Why You Die

The poison blocks messages from nerves to muscles. Within 10 to 45 minutes after dinner, numbness and tingling develop. Nausea, light-headedness, and a feeling of "impending doom" are commonly reported. Salivation, sweating, chest pain, difficulty swallowing and speaking, convulsions, and hypotension may result. Paralysis, difficulty breathing, and a decline in heart rate precede death. Some survivors have reported being paralyzed but totally alert, and one wonders if the dead experienced the same phenomenon while waiting to pass on.

To Live

If you ate the fish in the previous three hours, vomiting up the fish has a beneficial effect. But life-saving intervention usually requires rapid evacuation to a medical facility.

Moral: A great chef is worth the money.

81

RUBBED OUT BY RED TIDE

This fell sergeant, Death, is strict in his arrest.
WILLIAM SHAKESPEARE, 1600 OR SO

As sea currents bring in denser, cooler wedges of water from offshore, seeds of dinoflagellates are stirred up from their rest on the seafloor. These micro-algae are then exposed to enough sunlight and warm surface temperatures to bloom. They live through a single reproductive cycle and drop new seeds to the bed of the ocean to await another shift in the restless sea. These unicellular planktons are the foundation of the food chain, ranking second in abundance only to diatoms.

Inside the cell of a limited number of dinoflagellates, called *Alexandrium catenella*, toxins are produced. The most common encountered in the United States is saxitoxin. It is odorless, colorless, and tasteless. If the concentration of these dinoflagellates is high enough, they color the ocean: red tide. But a red tide does not have to occur for the dinoflagellates to be present in toxic numbers.

Many birds and fish are killed by the red blooms, but many shellfish (oysters, clams, mussels, scallops) store the toxins in their gills and digestive organs while suffering no ill effect. If you eat a "bad" shellfish, raw or steamed, the result could be paralytic shellfish poisoning.

Why You Die

Shortly after consumption, tingling starts in your lips and mouth. You won't have to wait long for abdominal cramping, nausea, vomiting, diarrhea, light-headedness, headache, difficulty with your vision, incoherence, and loss of coordination due to a creeping paralysis. If the paralysis creeps far enough, you'll lose the ability to breathe and retire forever to that oyster bed in the sky.

To Live

Drink a couple of glasses of water mixed with activated charcoal, and head for a hospital ASAP. If you stop breathing, rescue breathing may keep you alive. If your heart stops, CPR might keep you viable until you reach the hospital.

Moral: Clam up before it's too late.

82   SCORNED BY SCUBA

Man imagines that it is death he fears; but what he fears is the unforeseen, the explosion.

ANTOINE DE SAINT-EXUPÉRY, 1942

"Scuba" has been used as a stand-alone word for so long that many people have forgotten it is an acronym for "self-contained underwater breathing apparatus," originally an invention of Jacques Cousteau. Scuba divers breathe air that has been highly compressed into a tank. The air is fed to the diver through a regulator that regulates the pressure of the air being inhaled. As the diver descends underwater, air pressure increases dramatically, doubling at 33 feet, but the pressure of inhaled air from the tank remains the same. Everything works fine as long as the diver does not stay down too long, does not come up too fast—and remembers to keep breathing.

A diver who stays down too long or comes up too fast often has the nitrogen in the air being breathed form bubbles inside his or her body. The bubbles put pressure on tissues and cause pain. This is called "the bends" because bending (flexing) joints increases the pain. Death is rare, but permanent paralysis is not exceedingly rare.

Why You Die

If you are a diver who forgets to keep breathing, who holds your breath, you can have a serious problem if you ascend at the same time. This happens most often when you forget to check the gauge—and run out of air. The air inside your chest starts to increase in size as the ambient air pressure decreases on ascent. The increase in the space air takes up in your chest can cause injury from a depth as shallow as 4 feet. Suddenly your chest will explode. Not your chest, exactly, but parts of your lungs pop, making it very difficult to breathe. Air bubbles can enter your bloodstream through the rips and then enter your brain, causing a stroke-like death within minutes.

To Live

Never dive alone. A partner can share air. If alone, leave your regulator in your mouth. The air might expand enough on ascent to provide another breath. Look up as you ascend to keep your airway open, and keep exhaling slowly, very slowly.

> Moral: The secret of a long life
> is to keep breathing.

83 SILENCED BY SEA SNAKE

Sunset and evening star, and one clear
call for me! And may there be no moaning
of the bar, when I put out to sea.

ALFRED, LORD TENNYSON, 1889

Sea snakes, each and every one of the approximately 50 species, are venomous. Members of the family Hydrophiidae, they live almost exclusively in the western Pacific and Indian Oceans. One exception is the yellow-bellied sea snake, whose range includes the entire Pacific Ocean to the coast of Mexico and south. They average 4 to 6 feet in length, and some species may reach 10 feet or more. Air breathers, they must return to the surface regularly in order to survive. Living their lives in a liquid medium, however, has produced adaptations unique in the snake world. Slender and round in the front half, they flatten toward the rear into a paddle-like tail that allows them to swim with great finesse and to strike with agility by "springing" off their tails. Packing a virulent nerve toxin, sea snakes are among the most poisonous of creatures. While they vary in toxicity, at least one species has venom rated as 50 times more potent than that of a king cobra (see "Clobbered by Cobra"). Their fangs are like a cobra's, short and fixed, hollow and relatively small. They prefer to bite and consume small fish, but they bite humans, too, usually when they are accidentally handled or stepped on in shallow water.

Why You Die

Most victims report little pain, and most sea snake venom is relatively slow acting, although symptoms may appear in some cases within minutes. Within hours, surely, you'll feel growing anxiety, muscle stiffness, and muscle aches. The pain grows. Spastic paralysis follows. Nausea and vomiting typically complicate your remaining hours, which are often further characterized by restlessness, loss of bowel control, and deep unhappiness. Just before your ability to breathe fails, you'll have difficulty seeing. But heck, you'll have little interest in looking at anything by that time.

To Live

Wrap the bite site and the entire extremity on which it appears in an elastic bandage, but not tight enough to cut off circulation. Do not remove the bandage until you have arrived at a medical facility that has the antivenin.

Moral: A silent sea is not necessarily a safe sea.

SWALLOWED BY SPERM WHALE

Death is one moment, and life
is so many of them.

TENNESSEE WILLIAMS, 1963

Whales, the gentle giants of the sea, have little wish to cross paths with humans, largely due to the fact that humans have hunted and killed them for hundreds of years. Yet even when threatened, whales rarely cause harm to humans, and those rare times are often by accident. Sperm whales (*Physeter catodon*), growing to 60 feet in length, occasionally produce what some experts refer to as a "rogue male," documented to batter ships and drown seamen—and even less often to swallow humans.

In February of 1891 the whaling ship *Star of the East* harpooned a sperm whale in the South Atlantic, about 200 miles east of the Falkland Islands. Young James Bartley, on his apprentice voyage, was thrown from the longboat when the maddened whale beat the sea to froth. He disappeared. Whale's blood had attracted a congregation of sharks, and Bartley was given up as shark food. The whale eventually floated to the surface, dead, and was tied to the side of the ship and slowly butchered. When the whale's stomach was thrown aboard, it jumped as if alive. Bartley was removed from the stomach.

Why You Die

It would happen to you, most likely, as it supposedly happened to young James. He flopped on the deck, still breathing, bleached white of skin and hairless, blind, and unconscious. Approximately 15 hours had elapsed since the young man's disappearance. He lived more than long enough to return to England and tell his tale of falling into the whale's mouth, of screaming as he washed over the rows of tiny sharp teeth, of sliding down a long slimy tube, of blissful oblivion in the belly of the great mammal. Most people in this condition would, of course, have passed on from lack of air and/or from being dissolved in whale stomach acid.

To Live

Cold seawater was poured over James Bartley until he regained consciousness. It was weeks before his rational mind returned.

Moral: Some things are easier
to swallow than others.

The descent to Hades is much the same from whatever place we start.

ANAXAGORAS, FIFTH CENTURY BCE

If there be monsters in the sea, then they are probably giant squids, genus *Architeuthis*, which live way down deep, and whose length remains even today a source of debate, with estimates ranging from a mere 60 feet to a whopping 300 feet. To Norse of old they were called "kraken." To fishermen before the birth of Christ, they were feared as godless destroyers who rose to the surface after dark to drag down boats straggling in late toward shore. Frank W. Lane in his *Kingdom of the Octopus* says squid "are the most ferocious of all invertebrates."

In addition to their eight arms, squid have two long tentacles, which they shoot out with amazing speed to capture and haul in prey to their beaks for shredding and consuming. Distributed worldwide, they might rise to any surface of any ocean.

The passenger steamer *Strathowen*, crossing the Indian Ocean, on July 31, 1874, witnessed an attack on the *Pearl*, 150 tons of schooner: "Someone on the schooner fired a rifle at the (large brownish mass) and it began to move toward the schooner and squeezed on board between the fore and mainmast, pulling the vessel over and sinking it. Its body was as thick as the schooner and about half as long, with a train that appeared to be 100 feet long." The *Strathowen* picked up the survivors. The creature's tentacles, "which were as thick as a barrel," crushed a great many of the crew to death, and you can't say that about many dead people.

Why You Die
Other than being squished by the tentacles of a squid, you could, theoretically, be eaten. It is not known whether that has actually happened.

To Live
There appears to be only a slim chance you could struggle free of a giant squid's grasp, but it's worth a try.

Moral: Think twice before ordering calamari.

86

STABBED BY STINGRAY

I am not afraid to die. I just don't want
to be there when it happens.

WOODY ALLEN, *WITHOUT FEATHERS*

Rays, especially the large ones, soar gracefully through tropical and subtropical seas when on the move, but you can find several species swimming in freshwater. Divided into eight families and more than 500 species, they all fit into the order Myliobatiformes. Like sharks, they are boneless, and the flexible "wings" they soar with are actually wide fins. When hungry they sink to the bottom. Being flat and roundish, they are able to stir the sand on the ocean's floor to cover up while they wait for prey to pass by. They grab prey with their mouths.

Not all rays have stingers, but all stingrays do, and these barbed lances are used for defense, not for attacking. The stingers, one or two of them, grow fairly close to the base of their relatively long tails. If you happen to step on a stingray, which you might do since they like shallow water, most stingrays will think they are being attacked, and they will respond defensively.

Why You Die

Venom glands at the base of the stingers fill the stingers with poison that causes pain (a lot of it) and can cause death to the stung, usually via cardiac arrest. But, undoubtedly, the most famous death-by-stingray was Steve Irwin's. "The Crocodile Hunter" was pierced through the heart by a stingray's stinger, and he bled to death.

To Live

Wade in stingray-prone water with a shuffling step to avoid planting your foot on one. If you get stabbed, flush the wound with freshwater. Soaks in hot freshwater can ease the pain. Then wash the wound with soap and water. If your heart stops, hopefully someone nearby knows CPR and likes you.

Moral: Watch your step.

87

STUNNED BY STONEFISH

Death is the supple Suitor that wins at last . . .

EMILY DICKINSON, 1878

Inhabiting the seafloor in tropical waters, and occasionally in temperate waters, scorpion fish, family Scorpaenidae, sting with sharp spines that stick out of their backs like a row of poison-tipped nails. Some of the family members are lovely and graceful (lionfish, firefish, zebra fish) and carry a painful venom that produces ferocious pain. Some of these fish are exceedingly unattractive, lumps of flesh that resemble a part of the coral reef they call home more than a finned saltwater denizen. None of them is less appealing or more dangerous than stonefish (genus *Synanceja*), whose poison is rated by some as an equal to cobra venom.

If you inadvertently step on a stonefish, the most common way to make contact, one of the spines can easily puncture through sneakers or flippers, and pressure on the spine forces the venom up two paired ducts into your foot (or hand if you happen to reach for a stonefish). If provoked, stonefish have been known to attack.

Why You Die
Pain is immediate and immeasurably intense, but that's only the beginning. In 60 to 90 minutes, the pain will peak and stay peaked for 6 to 12 hours, pain cruel enough to drive the wimpy insane. Death in humans is fairly rare but often preferred by victims since it usually drops you in six to eight hours so you don't have to suffer so much. If you live, you'll have disconcerting stuff to look forward to in addition to the pain: headache, rash, nausea, vomiting, diarrhea, stomach pain, heavy sweating, arm and leg paralysis, fever, delirium, and seizures, to name a few of the better-known effects.

To Live

Soaking your hurting foot or hand in very hot water reduces the effects of the poison. Be sure to pick off anything that looks like part of a fish. If you get sick, antibiotics will probably be recommended, and antivenin for stonefish stings can sometimes be found in areas where stings are common.

Moral: You can learn things even from what appears to be a stone.

88

SLICED BY SURGEONFISH

Time gives the promise of time in
every death, not of any ceasing.

CHRISTOPHER FRY, 1956

Depending on whom you talk to, there are about 80 species of surgeonfish (family Acanthuridae) living mostly on or near tropical coral reefs. Many are brightly and beautifully colored, making them popular in saltwater aquariums, and most of them are on the small side, seldom growing to more than a foot or so in length, excepting the whitemargin unicornfish (*Naso annulatus*), largest of the surgeonfish, which grows to over 3 feet. All of them, however, grow one or two keenly sharp spines on both sides, scalpel-like things located where the body joins the tail, and they are not the least bit timid about using them. In some species the scalpels are fixed, and in others they are erectable. Tangs, another name for surgeonfish, can be territorial, and anytime they feel threatened they can and will slice out with fury and accuracy.

Why You Die

Even smaller species have nearly cut fingers from humans. The lacerations they make tend to be deep and painful, and your blood will flow freely. If it flows too freely, you will bleed to death. Bleeding divers have attracted much larger fish, namely sharks (see related entries in this book), and that

Death by Aquatic Accident

might count as a human killed by a surgeonfish if you are being generous to the tang.

To Live

Don't mess with surgeonfish. If you do, and if you're in the sea, get out. You need to stop the bleeding with direct pressure on the wound. The pain often persists. It will not kill you, but soaking the wound in hot water may ease the pain. With a big wound, find a doctor since infections, sometimes dangerous, are common.

> Moral: Surgeries are best performed in an operating room—with you asleep.

89

TORN APART BY TIGER SHARK

> We dread life's termination as the close,
> not of enjoyment, but of hope.
>
> WILLIAM HAZLITT, 1817

Sharks appeared before dinosaurs and have managed to thrive for about 350 million years. They circle the globe, preferring tropical and subtropical seas but being well documented to swim north to the Arctic. They have been caught as deep as 9,000 feet, and probably live even deeper. Without bones, they are made of stout and flexible cartilage, covered by incredibly rough skin, and teeth, lots of teeth, teeth that are soon replaced should one fall out, sharp teeth powered by monstrous jaw muscles. With an almost supernatural ability to sense prey, sharks can detect blood in water at as little as one part per million. Small of brain, large and voracious of appetite, sharks kill lots of things, and humans, although not a favored food of sharks, are by no means excepted.

Tiger sharks (*Galeocerdo cuvier*) develop faded darker gray vertical stripes on their lighter gray bodies and grow to 14 feet. The tiger shark is the largest shark on Pacific reefs and is also often seen from South Carolina southward and in the Bahamas. It is easily cataloged as one of the species most dangerous to humans: Ravenous hunger and poor eyesight have sent them after humans as food numerous times. Ravenous hunger and poor eyesight, in fact, have sent them after metal, wood, leather, and plastic, giving tiger sharks the nickname of "garbage can of the deep." They seem to prefer birds and turtles for food, but these sharks will consume anything the sea provides, more often feeding at night in shallow waters.

Why You Die
Keenly serrated, the teeth of a tiger shark tend to raggedly tear off parts of you after the shark bites and as it shakes its head. Your blood loss will be immediate and immense. After swallowing, the tiger shark will return for another bite. Soon a red smear delicately shading the water will be all that's left of you.

To Live
If you find yourself in the water with a shark, do not make rapid movements. If it attacks, strike the snout, eyes, and gills, preferably with something more substantial than your hand. If it bites you . . . well, best wishes.

> Moral: In the water at day, usually okay;
> in the water at night, shark's delight.

DEATH BY POISONOUS PLANT

Plants cannot run and hide. They can't "fight back," in the truest sense of that term, although some species protect themselves with thorns and sharp spikes. They mean no harm; they are simply trying to survive. In order to survive out there in this animal-eats-vegetation world, however, the most common defense mechanism of plants is not pointy but poisonous. Hundreds of species own a chemical. These chemicals range from mildly irritating to severely toxic. Here are some of the most deadly.

To be or not to be: that is the question.
WILLIAM SHAKESPEARE, AROUND 1600

Seven species of flowering plants in the genus *Brugmansia* are commonly called angel's trumpet. They grow fragrant and pendulous (hanging down) blooms that resemble, of course, trumpets—trumpets that may be 20 inches long and 14 inches across at the opening, the part where the sound would come out if they were real musical instruments. The flowers can be pink, red, orange, yellow, white, or green. The plants may be a shrub or a tree that reaches 36 feet in height, and they are native to the tropical regions of South America. In parts of America they are grown in gardens and around lawns as ornamentals, except where planting them is illegal due to the fact that all parts of the plant are poisonous, especially the seeds and leaves.

In some countries the leaves are steeped for a tea with the power to produce violent hallucinations. Be warned the hallucinations are not pleasant for most people, and drinkers have cut off important parts of their bodies under the influence, and, therefore, angel trumpet tea is not recommended. This plant is related to jimsonweed (see "Jinxed by Jimsonweed"), another un-recommended hallucinogenic.

Why You Die

The alkaloids in angel's trumpet may cause your pupils to dilate quickly. That's not a big deal, unless you have to drive somewhere, but then your heart will speed up, your head will hurt, you will suffer diarrhea, your body temperature will rise, and your smooth muscles will stop working. When the smooth muscles that run your lungs stop working, you cannot breathe—thus you die.

To Live

If you get to a medical facility in time, doctors will probably pump your stomach. If you arrive too late for that, you may get a drug called physostigmine, if they have it, which sometimes reverses the bad stuff. Here's the best idea: Do not consume any part of an angel's trumpet.

Moral: Blow your horn, not your mind.

91

BATTERED BY BANEBERRY

Death is not the opposite of life,
but an innate part of it.

HARUKI MURAKAMI, 2006

Avoiding anything named "bane" certainly seems like a fine idea. Within the genus *Actaea* there are at least two dozen species, but with the white baneberry (*Actaea pachypoda*) avoidance is especially recommended. Native to the eastern side of North America, this plant grows to about 2 feet high and 3 feet across with toothed leaves and small white spring flowers. What will stick in your mind, though, are the white berries at the end of reddish stems. At the rounded end of each berry a black spot makes the fruit look very much like the plant's nickname: doll's eye. It's a creepy doll's eye, a Chucky-ish eye. All parts of the plant contain poison, but the eyes abound with it. Half a dozen berries will make you very sick, and more will likely make you go bye-bye forever.

Why You Die

One reason you will die can be blamed on a lack of taste buds. These berries taste really awful: acrid, bitter. Why did you eat a second one? They contain a toxin that immediately attacks the heart. The sedative effect on cardiac muscle is acute. Soon you'll also experience a burning sensation in your mouth and throat followed by a headache, diarrhea, dizziness, and maybe hallucinations. Then your heart will arrest.

To Live

Don't ever eat a white berry. If you did within the hour, make yourself vomit. Then, if you happen to have some, swallow activated charcoal. Keep drinking water as you make your way ASAP to a doctor's place of business.

Moral: The eyes have it.

92

CRUCIFIED BY CASTOR BEAN

Life without knowledge is death in disguise.
TALIB KWELI, NOT LONG AGO

According to Guinness—the World Records and beer people—*Ricinus communis*, the castor bean, is the deadliest of all poisonous plants. It is widespread in tropical regions (the plant cannot deal with cold), with an alarming number of gardeners growing it for ornamental value. Unfortunately, different varieties of the plant assume different looks. No description will meet all identification needs. But all the plants bear fruit in the form of a capsule containing a large, oval, shiny seed. All the seeds, which are bean-like but not a true bean, contain a toxin called ricin.

Yes, the seeds are pressed into harmless and questionably useful castor oil, but chomped and swallowed raw it takes only four to eight seeds to bring death to a human—or just about any animal that eats them. Worth noting is this: If you swallow a seed whole, it probably won't hurt you. Some chewing is required.

Why You Die

Usually, after two to four hours, maybe longer, your mouth and throat will start to burn. Then expect abdominal pain, vomiting, and bloody diarrhea. Serious dehydration leads to a severe drop in blood pressure. When your blood pressure gets too low, your heart stops. The whole fatal process should be over in three to five days.

To Live

If you get to a hospital in time, the sooner the better, you have an excellent chance of being saved.

> Moral: Chewing your food well is
> not always the best idea.

93

DISTRESSED BY DEADLY NIGHTSHADE

Beauty is feared, more than death.

WILLIAM CARLOS WILLIAMS, 1948

Before America figured out it wanted to be a separate and therefore quite distinctive country, *Atropa belladonna*, a member of the widespread and numerous nightshade family (which includes the tomato), came over from Europe for a visit and decided to stay. Bell shaped and crowded on short branches with many leaves, the reddish, yellowish-green, or brownish-purple blooms are still considered of ornamental quality and grown on purpose by some gardeners. *Belladonna* means "beautiful lady" in Italian. Like many early Americans, these plants escaped the confines of civilization and now grow wild, especially in the East. Although the flowers and leaves, and even the roots, contain poisonous alkaloids, it's the fruit when it ripens to a bright black or purplish-black berry (up to a half inch across) that can kill, sometimes rather quickly. As few as three berries have been known to end the life of a small child.

Why You Die

As the alkaloids begin to take effect, you'll feel dry in the mouth and have a bit of difficulty swallowing. Your skin will grow warm and look pink, your heartbeat will quicken, your pupils will dilate, and you will have trouble seeing clearly. You may find it difficult to pee. You'll feel a sense of inexplicable excitement as your blood pressure rises and your heartbeat becomes erratic. Your mind will wander into delirium and confusion. As you slip into a coma, a sense of tranquility will pervade, from which comes the name "nightshade." Your respiratory drive will progressively fail,

to the point where you stop breathing forever.

To Live

From *Atropa belladonna* come the useful and common drugs atropine and scopolamine. From the beauty of her flowers comes a touch of the sublime. As a wine, deadly nightshade ranks among the last fluids you'll want in your stemware. Look and admire the Beautiful Lady, but don't touch. If you fail to follow this advice, hospitals usually have an antidote.

Moral: Beauty is only skin deep.

94 DEVASTATED BY DUMB CANE

Every soul will taste death.

QUR'AN (AL-IMRAN 3:185)

At least 56 species of the genus *Dieffenbachia* proliferate in tropical regions of the Western Hemisphere. Look for it in Mexico, over to the West Indies, and down to Argentina. Its showy, green, broad leaves speckled with attractive white splotches and its tolerance of shade make it popular as a house plant. What makes it unpopular are the needle-shaped and needle-sharp crystals, called raphides, within the cells of the leaves. (They are also in the roots and stems.) When chewed, an acute response in a human mouth to the raphides is a temporary loss of the power of speech. Since you can't speak, the plant deserves its common name of "dumb cane." It can do more than make you dumb.

Why You Die

After a brief bit of mastication, and a temporary bout of pretty severe oral burning, your mouth will go numb and you will start drooling. Frankly, the bad things often stop there. If not, your lips, mouth, throat, and tongue will start to swell. Oral blisters could form. If your tongue swells too much, you cannot get air in.

To Live

Death by dumb cane gets a rating of "rare" from experts. But since "rare" does not mean "never," find a doctor.

Moral: Dumb is as dumb does.

95

JINXED BY JIMSONWEED

Wisdom says: "We must die," and
seeks how to make us die well.

MIGUEL DE UNAMUNO, 1924

Especially in California and among the Southwestern tribes, shamans supposedly brewed a tea of jimsonweed (*Datura stramonium*), or a similar *Datura* species, and sipped their way into an altered state of consciousness in which secrets of the spirit world were revealed. History does not reveal how many shamans became permanent spirit world residents via jimsonweed, but you can rest assured that the whole plant, especially the roots, leaves, and seeds, contains hyoscyamine, a poison of the highest quality, a doorway to death through which many humans have passed.

Jimsonweed is a lush green plant at maturity, and the juices and wilted leaves hold the most toxin—as soldiers sent to Jamestown, Virginia, in 1666 discovered when they ran out of food and ate the berries and collapsed by the score. From Jamestown weed the name was corrupted to jimsonweed, also called Devil's trumpet (the white or purple flowers are trumpet shaped), stinkweed (it doesn't smell great), thorn apple (the berries are prickly), and mad apple (if you survive a sampling, you may report unpleasant hallucinations).

Why You Die

What you can expect several hours after consumption includes headache, dizziness, thirst (which can be extreme), a dry burning feeling in your skin, dilated pupils and a corresponding blurring of vision, perhaps blindness, delirium and manic activity, drowsiness, a weak pulse, a few seizures, coma, and very likely death. Some experts claim jimsonweed causes more poisonings than any other plant in the United States.

To Live

Avoid jimsonweed. In fact, avoid consuming, in any manner, any plant you cannot positively identify as safe. If avoidance fails, an antidote exists for jimsonweed and its relatives, and it might work.

> **Moral:** Some trips are worth the cost—and some aren't.

96

MISGUIDED BY MANCHINEEL

Death surprises us in the midst of our hopes.

THOMAS FULLER, 1732

Old Carib Indians dipped their arrowheads in the juice in case their aim failed to reach a vital organ. Clive Cussler splashed it in the beef Wellington to knock off almost the entire passenger list of an airline flight in *Treasure*. Early explorers, shipwrecked sailors, and typical tourists have succumbed to the sweet-tasting, crabapple-sized, and crabapple-shaped manchineel (*Hippomane mancinella*), the "death apple," growing in the Caribbean and around the Gulf of Mexico, including southern Florida's coastal hammocks.

Look for a tree that may grow to nearly 50 feet in height with rough, warty bark and shiny, oval leaves. The flowers may be yellow or red, giving way to light green or yellow fruit. The sap is milky. If you loaf beneath the leaves in a rain, water dripping onto your skin will give you a severe rash, probably within 30 minutes. Rub your rain-washed or sap-soaked finger in your eye and temporary blindness results. Toss the branches in a campfire and the smoke is likely to produce a headache and wickedly uncomfortable eye irritation.

Why You Die

Eating the tasty fruit (or the leaves) is a dead giveaway. One to two hours later, your lips, mouth, and throat will swell, burn, and blister. Stomach pain will be followed by vomiting and bloody diarrhea. Your pulse will soar and your breathing rate will follow. Your blood pressure will drop, and your face will drop to the ground, and before too awfully long your body will be pushing up manchineel.

To Live

If it touches your skin, wash immediately with soap and water. If you eat manchineel, find a doctor ASAP. There is no antidote, but medications to keep your blood pressure up have worked.

Moral: Sweetness ain't necessarily goodness.

> One must take all one's life to learn how to live,
> and, what will perhaps make you wonder more,
> one must take all one's life to learn how to die.
>
> SENECA, FIRST CENTURY CE

Throughout the Northern Hemisphere in temperate areas, you'll find a perennial herbaceous plant—actually several species in genus *Aconitum*—with attractive, dark blue monk's-hood–shaped flowers, pointy palmate leaves, and a vivacious poison lurking in the whole plant, especially the leaves and roots. Because they look edible, the roots have been mistaken for wild radish and consumed by humans, and the leaves have been tossed in salads. Monobasic alkaloids including aconine and aconitine can be ingested, when you eat monkshood, or absorbed, if the plant is rubbed on your skin. These poisons are most active before the plant flowers. Theoretically, you could persevere and rub enough into your skin to kill you, but you only have to eat very little of the plant for totally fatal results.

Why You Die
The early signs of your imminent death occur almost immediately: burning and tingling, maybe numbness, in the nose, throat, and face, followed quickly by nausea, vomiting, blurred vision, and a prickly feeling in your skin. Your

heartbeat will grow slow and weak, and you'll feel chest pain. Sweat will pour off you just before a series of convulsions set in. Numbness will spread over your entire body, and you'll feel cold from head to toe, as if your blood has been exchanged for ice water. Right behind numbness comes an unusual combination of paralysis and severe pain, which freezes your breathing muscles and your heart. Consciousness commonly prevails until the very end, and some victims have complained of "yellow-green vision" and ringing in the ears. Death has occurred in as little as 10 minutes.

To Live

No specific treatment works all the time, but magnesium sulfate has been used at least once with success. Doctors will keep you hydrated and provide supportive care, and hope for the best.

> **Moral:** Wear caution, and leave
> the hoods to the monks.

MISLED BY MUSHROOM

Death is the supreme festival
on the road to freedom.
DIETRICH BONHOEFFER, 1953

In Europe they once upon a time (and maybe still do) followed their pigs into the forest and gathered the mushrooms the pigs found. Pigs can sniff out a good mushroom before it breaks ground and avoid bad ones. But bad fungi erupt worldwide, and none rank as high among the potentially lethal as certain of the genus *Amanita* (deadly amanita, death cup, death cap, white amanita, destroying angel), which are responsible for approximately 90 to 95 percent of all deaths by mushroom.

Look for a chalky white mushroom with a bulbous base, up to 9 inches high and 4 to 6 inches across the white or yellowish-green to greenish-brown cap when mature, growing across the extent of the United States and Canada except on the Pacific Coast. Look for a veil hanging down like a shirt beneath the cap. Look for white or pale gills on the underside of the cap. Look for a mushroom even a pig won't eat.

Why You Die

After a meal of deadly mushroom, you'll feel fine for 6 to 24 hours. Then the complex polypeptides in the 'shroom suddenly produce severe abdominal cramps, profuse puking, watery diarrhea, blurred vision, and terrific thirst. Often the symptoms disappear, appear, and disappear again for periods of time. Don't be misled. The symptoms will usually return one last time, with prostration, coma, and death ensuing, usually within 48 hours. And even if you survive, which sometimes happens, your liver, kidneys, and heart may never be the same.

To Live

Do not eat a mushroom unless you are absolutely sure it is safe. If you know you ate a bad mushroom, make yourself vomit immediately after ingestion. Otherwise, find a doctor who will know best what to do.

Moral: Pick your mushrooms
at the grocery store.

99   OFFED BY OLEANDER

A dead man is nothing more than a dead man,
and a living man of the slightest pretensions
is stronger than the dead man's memory.

NAPOLEON I, ABOUT 1804

Native to the Mediterranean and Asiatic regions, oleander (*Nerium oleander*) has been imported to the United States for its ornamental qualities. It is a tall shrub, reaching 18 to 20 feet, and mildly fragrant. The leaves are lance shaped and leathery, the seed pods long and slender, the seeds hairy, and the flowers clustered at the ends of the branches in showy red, white, or pink. Oleander is one of the deadliest plants in the world. Its vibrant poisons include the cardiac glycosides oleandrin and nerioside, with actions similar to digitalis and with few equals in the vegetable realm. If eaten, a single leaf can off a full-grown adult. Children have succumbed after sucking the nectar from a single flower. Death has taken humans who ate hot dogs impaled and roasted on an oleander branch, or inhaled the smoke from branches thrown into a campfire, or ingested honey made from the juice of oleander flowers. Death has taken horses who ate the leaves, and the plant is called "horse killer" in some parts of the world and "ass killer" in others. Goats, for what it's worth, seem immune.

Why You Die

Almost immediately you'll experience nausea, followed by stomach pain and severe vomiting. Watch for bloody diarrhea, which should begin in a few hours. You'll feel cold and dizzy, and your heart will slow down and beat irregularly. Drowsiness and unconsciousness will precede a few convulsions and slow paralysis of your ability to breathe. Your death should occur in less than a day.

To Live

If you consumed the plant recently, try to make yourself vomit. You may take activated charcoal to absorb the poison. Some drugs have proven helpful in maintaining life, but they should be administered only under a doctor's supervision.

Moral: Wake up and smell the oleander.

100

RUN DOWN BY ROSARY PEA

Judge if you want, we are all going to die.
I intend to deserve it.

ANONYMOUS

Known by two dozen or so common local names (rosary pea, prayer bead, crab's eye, love pea, coral bead, and gidee gidee being some of them), *Abrus precatorius* grows as a native in India. But its capacity to eagerly invade tropical and subtropical regions, including Florida, has spread it around the globe. A slender woody vine, it twines around trees, bushes, shrubs, and hedges, and where it grows its fame follows due to two attributes of the seeds: Usually red with a black spot, they (1) make great beads, and (2) contain one of earth's most potent plant poisons. The Sunshine State has tagged the rosary pea Florida's Most Dangerous Plant.

The toxin is abrin, and when ingested it causes the victim to respond similarly to someone who has eaten a castor bean (see "Crucified by Castor Bean"). As with a castor bean, the seed has to be chewed, not just swallowed, to have ill effects. But just one rosary pea seed has been known to kill an adult human in as few as 36 hours.

Why You Die

Abrin prevents your cells from making protein, so they curl up and die. It works its bad stuff more slowly than many poisons.

You could start feeling nauseated and start vomiting in as few as 8 hours, but it could take as long as 3 days. A convulsion might be in your future. After several more days you will feel run down, your liver and/or other organs will fail, and you will pass on.

To Live

No antidote exists but supportive care, the kind you get in a hospital, gives you a pretty good chance of surviving.

Moral: Count your blessings, not your beads.

101

SNUFFED BY SNAKEROOT

Death is the last intimate thing we ever do.
LAURELL K. HAMILTON, 2000

They say, yes they do, Abe Lincoln's mother died of milk sickness. What that means is this: She drank enough milk from a cow that had eaten enough white snakeroot (*Ageratina altissima*) to cause the milk to be poisonous. Or maybe she ate enough beef from the cow. Either way can be fatal to humans. Before the plant's toxicity was identified, thousands of early immigrants to America perished in a manner similar to Ms. Lincoln's. Sometimes the cow died, too, as well as a bunch of sheep and horses. And that explains why white snakeroot appears on almost everybody's list of the 10 most deadly plants.

It is an herb of central and eastern North America with flat-topped clusters of small white flowers. The plant may reach 5 feet in height with leaves that can reach 7 inches long and grow in opposing pairs. It likes woodsy areas and brushy thickets. But you will not see white snakeroot so often these days since it is recognized and eradicated whenever possible.

Why You Die

Humans rarely eat the plant because it tastes terrible. Tremetol is the poison in the leaves and stems of the plant, and apparently animals don't find it so nasty to consume, and the poisoned animal, and its milk, don't taste bad to humans. You'll feel weak, you might start to tremble, you'll vomit, and your stomach will hurt a lot. If you ate enough, you'll slip into a coma that may last until your brain stops working.

To Live

No cure exists, but good supportive care in a fine medical facility often proves lifesaving.

Moral: Soy milk has a lot going for it.

102 SUCKED DOWN BY SUICIDE TREE

Death is the wish of some, the relief
of many, and the end of all.

SENECA, AROUND 60 CE

If it works for suicide, logic strongly suggests, and justifiably so, it works for murder, too. Despite logic, *Cerbera odollam* is called the suicide tree and a host of other names (such as famentana, pong-pong, kisopo, and othalanga), but it is nowhere called the murder tree. On the other homicidal hand, the toxin in this plant shows up rarely in autopsies, and thus it has been called an almost perfect murder weapon. Murders aside, researchers, who shall remain herein unnamed, state with almost absolute certainty that no other plant has been used more often by humans to take their own lives. Most of them, the trees, grow in India. You can find them here and there in other places in southern Asia, and most often rooted in salty swamps and marshy areas. They are related to and bear a strong resemblance to oleander (see "Offed by Oleander"). The suicide tree, a hardwood, can grow to over 30 feet tall, with long pointed leaves like a lance's tip, but it is the fruit, looking much like young mangos, that contains the poisonous seeds. The fruit, by the way, tastes bitter, but not bitter enough to deter occasional accidental sampling.

Why You Die

Seeds of the suicide tree contain toxins, cerberin primarily, that disrupt the normal activity of your heart muscle. Within hours you may experience abdominal pain, diarrhea, vomiting, and an irregular heart rhythm. If you have consumed enough of the toxin, your heart stops beating altogether. "Enough," a commonly relative term, here can mean as few as one seed.

To Live

Depending on how much cerberin you ate, you may have a day or two to live. As soon as possible, therefore, get your stomach pumped. If you act soon enough, you will likely rid yourself of a lethal wallop of the bad stuff. Consuming large doses of potassium seems to counter the effects of the poison. It appears nothing else will help.

Moral: Suicide is a permanent solution
to a temporary problem.

Nobody knows, in fact, what death is, nor whether to man it is not perchance the greatest of all blessings; yet people fear it as if they surely knew it to be the worst of evils.

SOCRATES, CIRCA 399 BCE

Shortly after Socrates, the infinitely brilliant Greek philosopher, uttered two of the most important words ever uttered, "Know thyself," he was forced to drink tea brewed from *Cicuta maculata* or perhaps a related species, a plant called water hemlock. Apparently his innovative philosophies were deemed subversive by the state.

C. maculata grows, as you would expect, along the banks of waterways or in wet meadows throughout North America. It bears, in addition to hemlock, such names as children's bane, beaver poison, death-of-man, poison parsnip, and false parsley. A member of the parsnip or carrot family, it stands tall with hollow stems and a bundle of short rootstocks that exude an oily yellow juice when cut. Its leaves are alternate and pinnate with two to three leaflets that are narrow, toothed, and pointy. Its flowers are white and small, blossoming in flat-topped, umbrella-like clusters, like a carrot in bloom. The entire plant, but especially the roots and young plants in spring, is poisonous. A full-grown adult can be killed by one bite of root, and children have died from simply using the hollow stems as peashooters. The poison is resin-like cicutoxin, a toxin that acts on the central nervous system of the victim. Many death-by-plant experts consider water hemlock to be the most poisonous plant in the North Temperate Zone.

Why You Die

Within 30 minutes of consuming water hemlock, you will vomit and have a convulsion or two. You may feel better after puking, but the plant only lulls you into a false sense of security. Soon your heart rate will speed up, your pupils will dilate, and you'll sweat like you just ran a marathon in southern Georgia in July. You'll begin to froth at the mouth and jerk violently in severe seizures. You'll probably experience extraordinary stomach pain, vomit a time or two more, slip into delirium, and stop breathing for a few minutes now and then. Paralysis will take over, and soon you'll stop breathing forever.

To Live

Learn to recognize water hemlock and avoid all contact. There is no specific antidote. If you think you swallowed water hemlock, make yourself vomit immediately. Then swallow some activated charcoal ASAP and find a doctor.

Moral: Know thy water-related plants.

DEATH BY DISASTROUS DISEASE

The World Health Organization (WHO) currently says there are approximately 13,000 diseases available on this planet. Some of them are veiled in mystery and some of them seem to result from humans acting in unwise ways, such as inhaling tobacco smoke. Most of them, however, get a grip on humans via pathogens (germs that cause disease). Germs fall generally into four categories: ultra-tiny viruses (16,000 could fit on the head of a pin), bacteria (single-cell organisms that move through life on the whims of nature), protozoa (single-cell organisms with the ability to move themselves), and fungi (multi-cell organisms that decompose material and live off the decomposition). Many germs can cause death.

104

CRAMPED BY CONSTIPATION

Death either destroys or unhusks us.
If it means liberation, better things
await us when our burden's gone.

SENECA, FIRST CENTURY CE

Constipation is infrequent and/or difficult movement of the bowels usually created by either a fluid level too low to lubricate your tract or a fiber level too low to keep things rolling along, and it can be encouraged by poor exercise habits. You can also ignore the urge to go until your fecal matter hardens to the point where, when you do try, you feel like you're trying to push out a brick (which is sort of true). Humans ignore the urge fairly often in the wild outdoors, especially if they are not used to pooping in the woods. If your bowels don't move at least three times per week, says medical science, you're constipated—but individual differences do exist. If you haven't had a bowel movement in three days, you will typically feel crampy and uncomfortable. After five days you could be developing serious problems from the toxins building up in your intestinal tract. If you end up in the hospital, a not uncommon result, a doctor might feel the medical need to insert a finger or two to break up the blockage, and that fact has encouraged the sale of laxatives.

Why You Die

Admittedly, death by constipation is rare. But on those rare occasions, your intestines will be reabsorbing the toxins from decaying fecal matter and sharing them with the rest of your body.

To Live

Drink plenty of water (try for at least three quarts per day) and eat healthy. If you get constipated anyway, drink even more water, and eat lots of whole grains, fruits, and vegetables. Avoid peanut butter, cheese, and high-fat foods. Many people, to encourage movement, add a stool softener—preferably a suppository.

Moral: Yes, some people are full of s—t!

105

DOOMED BY DENGUE

Death is unstoppable. One must
face it as a fact of life.

D. ASWINI, 2013

Blame mosquitoes again. They, primarily *Aedes aegypti* mosquitoes, sometimes carry the dengue virus. Enough of them
carry it to infect probably more than 400 million humans in
tropical regions of earth every year. You don't get the disease
from another human. If you get bitten by an infected mosquito, you may not know it. Not all humans develop symptoms, and some develop only mild symptoms, usually a low
fever. Many thousands, however, grow ill with full-on dengue
fever: a high fever, a bad headache, vomiting, severe joint and
muscle pain, and a skin rash. If you get dengue fever, you'll
feel terrible for usually less than a week. Then you get well.
There is no specific cure, but you can improve your chances
of getting well with supportive care. While you're feeling terrible, drink plenty of fluids but do not take aspirin, ibuprofen,
or any other drug that encourages bleeding.

Why You Die

Statistics vary annually, but somewhere between 1 and 5 percent of dengue fever sufferers go on to develop and die from
dengue hemorrhagic fever or dengue shock syndrome. With
the first one you bleed until your circulatory system fails, and

with the second one your blood pressure sinks too low to sustain life.

To Live

No vaccine currently exists, so the only way to avoid the dengue virus is to avoid getting mosquito bitten (see "Murdered by Mosquito")—or stay away from the tropics.

> Moral: It is better to use a repellent
> than to be a repellent.

106

DRAINED BY DIARRHEA

I have asked for death. Begged for it. Prayed
for it. Then the worst thing can't be death.

ARCHIBALD MACLEISH, 1958

Tabor's Medical Dictionary describes it as "frequent passage
of unformed watery bowel movements." People who have a
bad case call it "worse than death," but they are probably
suffering the worse of two broad types of diarrhea. Invasive
diarrhea, from bacterial sources and sometimes called dysentery, attacks the lower intestinal wall, causing inflammation, abscesses, and ulcers that may lead to mucus and blood
(often "black blood" from the action of digestive juices) in
stools, high fever, "stomach" cramps from the depths of hell,
and significant amounts of body fluid rushing from the nether
region. The second type, noninvasive diarrhea, grows from
colonies of microscopic evildoers that set up housekeeping
on, but without invading, intestinal walls. Toxins released
by the colonies cause cramps, nausea, vomiting, and, again,
sometimes massive gushes of fluid from your lower intestinal tract. Diarrheal illnesses come and go with the vagaries
of what one voluntarily and involuntarily ingests; erupt from
numerous sources that include bacteria, viruses, and protozoa; and last as briefly as a relatively blessed six hours or as
long as a destructive three weeks or more.

Why You Die

Whatever the causative agent, a diarrheal illness can be mild, moderate, or severe depending on the frequency of the rush, the pain of cramping, the wateriness of the bowel movement, and the vileness of the gas—the latter being often a matter of personal opinion. All cases, however, have in common the departure of water from humanity's hindmost orifice—sometimes oceans of fluid, up to 25 liters in 24 hours in the most severe cases. The severe cases, causing death-dealing dehydration (see "Dried Out by Dehydration"), end more lives worldwide every year than any other secondary reason.

To Live

Replace the lost fluid. Clear liquids are the best choice, liquids such as plain water, broths, herbal teas, and fruit juices you can see through. If the illness continues, you will require additional electrolytes, especially sodium. Pepto-Bismol may relieve some of the torture of diarrhea, but stronger drugs should probably be withheld for 24 hours. When you choose stronger drugs, Imodium is often recommended by physicians. If the diarrhea persists for 24 to 72 hours, and especially if you think you have dysentery, find a doctor.

Moral: You are what you eat.

107

HUNG UP BY HANTAVIRUS

> Though it be in the power of the weakest
> arm to take away life, it is not in the
> strongest to deprive us of death.
>
> SIR THOMAS BROWNE, 1642

Carried in rodent urine, and probably in feces and saliva, hantavirus can become airborne through misting of urine or in dust from dried feces and nests. The virus has been found predominantly in deer mice but also in pinyon mice and chipmunks, and other small rodents probably carry it. So far no known transmission of the germs has occurred between insects and humans or between humans and humans. You will most likely inhale the germs after messing around in an old, rodent-infested outbuilding, or while you sleep on the ground near a nest, or if you camp sloppily and attract sick rodents to your campsite. The viral particles you breathe in take up residence in your lungs regardless of your age, weight, height, gender, or ethnic background.

Why You Die

The incubation period for hantavirus infection is usually somewhere between two and four weeks. You'll start with fever and muscle aches and think, rats, you've contracted some kind of flu. More symptoms develop that fail to alter your first self-diagnosis. You may have a cough, headache, abdominal pain, and sometimes itchy, inflamed eyes. But then, *wham*, you are hit by the sudden onset of adult respiratory distress syndrome, featuring fluid in your lungs and severe difficulty breathing that gets progressively worse until you can breathe no more. To date the infection has ended the life of one out of every three people who were diagnosed with it.

To Live

Get to a hospital as soon as possible. No specific treatment exists, but definitive medical attention gives you the best chance of survival.

Moral: Never rat on your friends.

108

LAID LOW BY LEPTOSPIROSIS

Death hath a thousand doors to let out life.

PHILIP MASSINGER, 1640

Members of an order of slender, spiral, microscopic organisms belonging to the class Schizomycetes, spirochetes of the genus *Leptospira* have hooked or curved ends, and leptospirosis is the disease these organisms cause once they get inside humans. Leptospirosis appears throughout tropical and temperate regions of the world and is most commonly seen in Southeast Asia and some areas of Latin America. Recent cases have been brought back to the United States from lower Central America.

Although infected wild animals, including some frogs and snakes, show no signs of the disease, they shed the spirochetes freely in their urine. Human cases, usually fewer than 100 each year in the United States, are most often acquired from contact with contaminated water, and sometimes contact with soil. Swallowing ranks as the primary way *Leptospira* get inside people, but the organisms can "worm" in through abraded skin and through the mucous membranes of the eyes and mouth. You can also get sick from contacting infected animal blood and tissues.

Why You Die

Numerous types of *Leptospira* exist, but the signs and symptoms they produce in humans are much the same. One to two weeks (it can be as long as three) after invasion of the spirochetes, the first of two phases of the disease begins. Phase one lasts four to seven days and shows up in many patients as fever, chills, headache, enlarged lymph nodes, malaise, and a nonproductive cough. After a couple of days off, the disease reappears in the second phase, causing a lower fever and a severe headache that won't go away. A spotty rash sometimes appears. Muscle aches, stomach pain, nausea, and vomiting can result in either or both phases. Death occurs about 5 percent of the time, most often in the very young and very old, when the organisms work their way into kidneys, liver, or heart.

To Live

Treatment is a rather involved process that includes antibiotics to kill the spirochetes and then the struggle against possible complications. You will require definitive medical aid.

Moral: Keep your mouth shut.

109

LICKED BY LYME DISEASE

You will not die because you are ill,
but because you're alive.

SENECA, FIRST CENTURY CE

Bacteria of the order Spirochaetales include *Borrelia burgdorferi*, a spiral-shaped organism, the cause of Lyme disease. The disease was first recognized in the area around Lyme, Connecticut, in 1975, and now at least 45 states believe it is transmitted by ticks in their area, the deer tick getting most of the blame. Lyme disease, or something very nearly Lyme disease, has cropped up in Europe, Asia, and Australia. The bacteria live in animals, deer mice being a huge reservoir, and the ticks feed on infected blood and then pass the disease to you if you happen to be around at the appropriate time—feeding time for the tick.

Why You Die

Lyme disease has three stages: (1) An average of seven days after the tick bite, many people develop a marvelous red rash with definite borders that appears in some areas of your body, then fades and reappears in other areas. The rash hangs around for an average of four weeks. (2) Malaise and fatigue start from days to weeks after the bacteria get inside you and can become severe. A low fever, muscle aches, and other signs and symptoms that you might associate with a "flu bug" manifest themselves. This can go on for weeks. (3) Your knees and other large joints start to ache with arthritis after about a year or so. But in fact it is very difficult to die from Lyme disease. You have to be cursed, and the bacteria have to work their way into your heart and cause a block in the impulses that keep your heart beating, and the block has to be severe enough to prevent it from being corrected.

To Live

With antibiotic treatment, started soon enough, the germs die. If you remove an embedded tick with tweezers by grabbing it gently near your skin and pulling straight out, and if you do this within 48 hours after the tick embeds, you will probably not get sick with Lyme disease. Remember, ticks prefer to embed in dark, warm, moist, embarrassing areas of your body. As many as one out of every four ticks embed somewhere you can't see on yourself!

> Moral: At tick check time you learn
> who your real friends are.

So, have a little fun. Soon enough you'll be dead
and burning in Hell with the rest of your family.

GEORGE CARLIN, 1998

Well over 200 million new cases of malaria will occur in humans this year, and this fact has been true for quite a large number of years. These humans got bit by a female *Anopheles* mosquito that had a parasitic protozoan of the genus *Plasmodium* in her saliva. In approximately four out of five victims of malaria, the disease rates as "uncomplicated": people get sick with flu-like symptoms, and then those people get well.

The other one out of five dies, usually in Africa, and usually, but certainly not always, because that human is a child. To be more precise, the number of people who die from malaria every year approaches half a million. For those who are interested, a case of serious malaria in the United States is "very rare."

Why You Die

Once in the human bloodstream, the parasites rush to the human liver, where they settle down, mature, and reproduce. Then the parasites spread through the body killing red blood cells. You can die from that. And you can die if the parasites take over your brain. And, probably worst of all, you can die if they take over your lungs: You'll put a great deal of effort into sucking in air, but you won't be able to suck in enough.

To Live

Antimalarial drugs, taken prophylactically, will kill the parasites in your body before you get sick. If you do get malaria, there are drugs that almost always make you well. You should also do your best to prevent getting bitten (see "Murdered by Mosquito").

Moral: Just say yes to some drugs.

111

PUT AWAY BY PLAGUE

I bet it was pretty hard to pick up
girls if you had the Black Death.

JACK HANDY, 1992

Between 1347 and 1350 the Black Death, caused by the bacterium *Yersinia pestis*, started in Asia and eventually rubbed out about 25 million Europeans (roughly one-third of the population), including nine-tenths of the people of England. Before those devastating years, even in BCE days, reports of the ravages of plague were known and feared.

Plague is carried by rodents and passed primarily by the bite of rodent fleas, and both rodent and flea are killed by the germs, an unusual aspect of this disease. Black rats are especially susceptible, and *Rattus rattus* is blamed for the Black Death. In the United States deer mice and various voles maintain the bacterium. It is amplified in prairie dogs and ground squirrels. Other suspects include chipmunks, marmots, wood rats, rabbits, and hares. States in which plague still exists include New Mexico, Arizona, California, Colorado, Utah, Oregon, and Nevada.

Hikers and campers in infected areas are at risk. Meat-eating pets that eat infected rodents (or get bitten by infected fleas) can acquire plague. Dogs don't get very sick, but cats do. Only one case of plague being passed to a human by a dog is known, but cats can pass the disease to humans by biting them, coughing on them, or carrying their fleas to them. In the wild coyotes and bobcats are known to have transmitted plague to humans after the critters were dead and the humans were skinning them. Skunks, raccoons, and badgers are suspect. Sick people transmit plague readily to other people.

Why You Die

Several forms of plague exist, but the three most common are bubonic, septicemic, and pneumonic. Buboes are inflamed lymph nodes, and they give bubonic plague its name. After an incubation period of two to six days, patients usually suffer fever, chills, malaise, muscle aches, and headaches. Blackened, bleeding skin sores gave a name to the Black Death. There's simply no way to look good while you're dying. The septicemic form may appear similar but does not give rise to buboes. Gastrointestinal pain with nausea, vomiting, and diarrhea is common. The pneumonic form results most often from inhaling droplets, but it can develop from bacteria that got into your blood. Coughing often produces blood in the sputum. With the infection in your blood and lungs, septicemic and pneumonic, respectively, your chances are slimmer than with the bubonic form. But all forms commonly overwhelm your body's ability to support life.

To Live

If you suspect plague, you should seek treatment with the appropriate drugs, after which life usually goes on. Prevention includes avoiding rodents, avoiding touching sick or dead animals, and restraining dogs and cats while traveling in infected areas.

Moral: Flee the flea.

RAVAGED BY RABIES

> Man is the only animal that contemplates
> death, and also the only animal that
> shows any sign of doubt of its finality.
>
> WILLIAM ERNEST HOCKING, 1957

By the 1990s two or fewer humans in the United States died from rabies every year, and what few infections did pop up were acquired from the bites of bats—but worldwide, rabies kills somewhere between 40,000 and 70,000 people every year. While it is often thought of as a disease of carnivores, any mammal can theoretically have rabies, and cows are the most common domestic animal to carry the disease. Despite the publicity mad dogs have received, rabid cats outnumber rabid dogs, with 290 infected cats being destroyed in a recent single year, compared to 182 infected dogs in the same year. Unfortunately, rabies in wild animals seems to be on the rise, with more than 50,000 infections identified in US raccoons since 1975. Skunks are also way up there in infections. Bats, raccoons, and skunks account, say some experts, for 96 percent of the rabies cases in wild animals of the United States. Foxes and coyotes make up most of the missing 4 percent. Foxes are the leading source of rabies in Europe; mongooses in Puerto Rico; dogs in Africa, South America, and most of Asia; and wolves and jackals in India and Israel.

Shaped like an ultramicroscopic bullet, the virus, carried in the saliva of infected animals, attaches itself to peripheral nerves at the bite site and moves slowly but with great determination along nerves toward the brain. Since rabies causes no reaction until it reaches the central nervous system, you don't know you're infected until it's too late. Once replication of the virus starts in the brain, nasty death invariably results. Before the death of the human host, the virus, after multiplying in neurons, moves back out along nerves and congregates in different body parts, including skin, corneas, and salivary glands, at which time the infected human can pass on the virus. Around BCE Mesopotamia, physicians first described the horror of dying from rabies. The agonizing difficulty in swallowing, sometimes caused by the mere sight of water, produced the common name of "hydrophobia," a fear of water.

Why You Die

Early symptoms of rabies are too general to cause concern: fatigue, headache, irritability, depression, nausea, fever, and stomach pain. Sounds like another day at the office. There is only one way to know for sure if you have the disease: You die! But first: wild hallucinations, including episodes of unexplainable terror; extremely painful difficulty swallowing, to the point where you refuse all liquids and drool constantly; frequent muscle spasms, especially in the face and neck; and toward the end, complete disorientation and a raging fever.

To Live

Vaccinations prior to exposure will prevent the disease if you get bitten. After a bite injections can kill the virus, if you get them before the germs reach your brain.

Moral: Never feed the mouth that bites.

113 SICKENED BY SALMONELLA

No one escapes from life alive.

MICHAEL CRICHTON, 1980

Many different types of *Salmonella* bacteria hang out on earth in domestic and wild animals. Some types you would see more often than others if you could see something that small, which you can't, but they make humans sick when they start hanging out in your intestines. The bacteria usually get into intestines by being consumed along with contaminated food or water. The food is most often undercooked meat, raw eggs, and sometimes dairy products, but any raw food could be bad. Salmonella can live for weeks in bad food and months in bad water. You can consume the germs easily by getting them on your hands and then using those hands to put uncontaminated food into your mouth. (If you have it in your gut, you will be pooping it out.) The disease, known as salmonellosis, will make about 1.2 million sick (with abdominal pain, diarrhea, and fever) in the United States over the coming year. Most of those people will say they have food poisoning, and somewhere between 400 and 500 will die. In other parts of the earth, without good medical care, the death rate, some years, reaches to more than 20 percent of those infected.

Why You Die

Since most sufferers do not die, your chances of surviving salmonellosis in the United States are excellent. The germs will probably stay in your gut, but they can migrate into your bloodstream and show up in vital parts, and those parts can stop working—and then so do you.

To Live

Cook all meats thoroughly. Wash all raw food before eating and, probably more important, wash your hands well before prepping food. In the wild outdoors use a water disinfection method that eliminates bacteria.

Moral: Dirty hands are the devil's tools.

114 SPACED OUT BY SPOTTED FEVER

> Life is strewn with so many dangers, and
> can be the source of so many misfortunes,
> that death is not the greatest of them.

NAPOLEON I, AROUND 1804

Transmitted by the bite of ticks, Rocky Mountain spotted fever is not limited to the Rocky Mountains, even though it was first diagnosed there; in fact, it appears all over the United States, with most cases having recently occurred in North Carolina and Oklahoma. Neither is it a fever with spots. It is a disease that gives you a spotty rash and a high fever. The cause is bacteria that live well inside of ticks, especially wood ticks and American dog ticks, a bacterium (*Rickettsia rickettsii*) of the family Rickettsiaceae, a bacterium that may live well inside of you. The ticks feed on any warm-blooded mammal. If the mammal has the bacteria, ticks pick up the organisms and pass them to you should they find your warm blood available at mealtime. RMSF is the most dangerous, the most lethal rickettsial disease in America.

Why You Die

The incubation period, the time from the tick bite until you know you're sick, can range from 2 to 14 days. Along with the sudden onset of fever, chills, headache, and muscle aches, you will develop a rash that spreads over your entire body, including the palms of your hands and the soles of your feet. You may also have stomach pain, vomiting, diarrhea, and confusion about what's going on. You have a fairly okay chance of surviving, but the bacteria invade the walls of your blood vessels, primarily your arteries and arterioles, and your heart muscle, and can collapse your vasculature within as little as six days of the tick bite. Untreated, about 3 out of 10 humans (or 30 percent) die from RMSF.

To Live

With antibiotic treatment the number of people who die from RMSF drops to somewhere between 3 and 5 percent annually. If embedded ticks are removed soon enough, they do not feed long enough to pass the disease.

Moral: Don't get ticked off, get the tick off.

115   TRAPPED BY TETANUS

Every tiny part of us cries out against the
idea of dying, and hopes to live forever.

UGO BETTI, 1949

Spores of hardy *Clostridium tetani* rank among the world's most common bacterial inhabitants of soil and vegetation. Approximately 1 out of every 10 humans carries the bacteria in his or her intestinal tract. When the germs get into an anaerobic environment, say, trapped in the bottom of a dirty wound, the spores germinate and release a toxin. This toxin, tetanospasmin, causes the disease tetanus, which has been recognized since the days of the medically oriented ancient Greeks. Mortality rates for tetanus, even today, approach 40 percent in adults and 90 percent in children. That's why even tiny babies are vaccinated against the disease.

Why You Die

The incubation period may run from 1 to 55 days, but symptoms tend to show up within two weeks. Tetanospasmin spreads throughout your nervous system, where it interferes with the production of inhibitory neurotransmitters, which means you start having violent muscular spasms. Rigidity of your jaw muscles (called trismus or lockjaw) with difficulty swallowing will usually be your first complaint. Expect signs of sympathetic nervous system involvement: rapid heart rate, sweating, and a rise in blood pressure. Seizures are common. Breathing may become difficult, and respiratory failure will probably be the eventual cause of your death.

To Live

Keep your tetanus immunizations up to date with a shot at least once every 10 years.

> Moral: Getting "needled" is not
> always a bad thing.

TRICKED BY TRICHINOSIS

> All human things are subject to decay, and
> when fate summons, monarchs must obey.
> JOHN DRYDEN, 1682

Encysted in skeletal muscle, the larvae of the parasitic round-worm *Trichinella spiralis* are eaten by some hungry eater of meat. In the small intestine the worms mature and mate within a few days, often within 48 hours. Female worms deposit larvae in nearby mucosal tissue. Larvae squirm into the lymphatic system and then the circulatory system of the animal and invade skeletal muscle. Within three weeks the larvae are encysted and ready to be infectiously passed should anything eat the muscle of the animal that ate the muscle of the animal that had encysted larvae.

Although all carnivorous and omnivorous mammals may have trichinosis, consumption of raw or undercooked pork accounts for the vast majority of the disease in humans. Rodents are often infected, but mice and rats seldom grace a human palate. Bears, raccoons, opossums, seals, walruses, peccaries, and wild swine are common hosts, and sometimes are eaten by humans.

Why You Die

Some people never know they have the worms inside them, but you may suffer gastrointestinal symptoms during the first week after ingestion of infected meat: pain, nausea, vomiting, and variable diarrhea. The severity of the symptoms depends on the number of larvae eaten. During the second week, as the larvae migrate around your body, capillary damage occurs, commonly producing facial edema and maybe producing hemorrhages in nail beds and the conjunctiva. Migrating larvae can invade the pulmonary system, causing a cough and chest pain, or the heart muscle, causing carditis and a chance at patient death. Gastrointestinal symptoms may remain for four to six weeks, until the worms are all excreted. As the larvae encyst in muscle tissue, significant muscle aches and stiffness often result. Between 6 and 18 months after ingestion, the larvae die and become calcified. This period is usually asymptomatic, and if you made it this far, you'll have to find another way to die.

To Live

Drugs can kill the adult worms, but nothing will kill the larvae. A doctor will know best what to do while you wait for fate to decide.

> **Moral:** Pigs can't swim and pigs can't fly,
> but pigs can sometimes make you die.

117

TORTURED BY TULAREMIA

Hardest of deaths to a mortal is
the death he sees ahead.

BACCHYLIDES, FIFTH CENTURY BCE

The Japanese physician Soken first spotted the disease in people who got sick from eating "bad" rabbit meat in the year 1837. Since 1967 fewer than 200 cases per year have been diagnosed in the United States. In 1912 the disease was isolated in rodents in Tulare County, California, and thus the sickness, caused by the coccobacillus *Francisella tularensis*, acquired its common name of tularemia.

Though tularemia was certainly once a disease associated with unhealthy contact with rabbits, ticks are now, by far, considered the prime transmission mode for the bacteria. Many species of ticks have been incriminated, but dog ticks and lone star ticks rank as the most common reservoirs. Since the infecting organisms have not been found in tick saliva, it is thought they are carried in tick feces. Rabbits still qualify as the second most common vector, but you must handle infected tissue, as you might do by skinning and eviscerating the little bunny. You could pick up the disease in water or soil, too, by direct contact, ingestion, or breathing in contaminated dust or water particles.

Why You Die

Most cases appear as a sudden onset of high fever and headache. About 80 percent of tularemia cases appear in an ulceroglandular form: red bumps harden and ulcerate, usually on the lower extremities where the ticks bit or on the hands from handling infected tissues. Ulcers are typically painful and tender. Enlarged tender lymph nodes are common. The second most common form of tularemia, the typhoidal form, causes fever, chills, and debility. Weight loss may be significant. Lymph node enlargement is less. Pneumonia is a relatively common complication of tularemia. If you can work up a serious pneumonia, you can increase your chances of dying from 5 percent to 30 percent.

To Live

Take every precaution to prevent being bitten by a tick. If you must handle dead animals, especially rabbits, wear gloves. If you get sick, find a doctor. Antibiotics almost always end the illness.

Moral: Let sleeping rabbits lie.

118

WILTED BY WEST NILE

Death borders upon our birth, and
our cradle stands in the grave.

JOSEPH HALL, 1608

Uganda, 1937: The first case of West Nile virus is officially identified. But no known case appeared in the United States until the summer of 1999. Since that first victim in the New York City area, the disease has been reported all across the country, the extreme Northeast and Hawaii excepted.

Mosquitoes seem to get the virus from infected birds and maintain it in their salivary glands—then spread it to humans when they bite and feed. West Nile virus has also been found in horses, cats, bats, chipmunks, squirrels, skunks, and domestic rabbits, but there is no evidence that humans get the virus from other animals, including other humans, without a mosquito serving as the go-between.

Fewer than one in five people who contract the disease develop any symptoms. If the signs and symptoms develop, they may take 3 to 14 days (5 to 15 days, say some experts) after inoculation, and they are almost always mild and flu-like. They may include fever, headache, muscle aches, and occasionally a rash on the trunk of the body and swollen lymph glands. These signs and symptoms eventually go away harmlessly, often within a few days.

Why You Die

In rare cases—approximately 1 in 150—the virus can cross the blood-brain barrier and cause a serious inflammation of the brain (known as West Nile encephalitis), a serious inflammation of the membranes surrounding the brain and spinal cord (known as West Nile meningitis), or a serious inflammation of the brain and its surrounding membranes (known as West Nile meningoencephalitis). Serious signs and symptoms may include headache, high fever, neck stiffness, stupor, disorientation, coma, tremors, convulsions, muscle weakness, and paralysis. In severe cases the problems may persist for weeks and the neurological effects may be permanent. In less than 0.1 percent of cases in the United States, the sick person dies.

To Live

A blood test can tell you if you are sick with West Nile virus. Unfortunately, there exists no specific treatment, but supportive care leads to a complete recovery in all but a few people.

> **Moral:** Your chances of being struck by lightning are slightly better than your chances of dying of West Nile virus.

DEATH BY NEFARIOUS NATURE

Okay, nature is not wicked or evil—unless you count as evil anything completely uncaring. Nature does not care about anything at all. But it does follow the rules. The rules include: A human has to have an almost constant flow of oxygen, a human must consume a certain number of calories, and a human must maintain a specific and rather narrow range of body core temperatures. Nothing explains with absolute certainty where the rules came from. Nature? But it is certain that breaking the rules can and often does cause death.

119

ALTERED BY ALTITUDE

> What is called a reason for living is
> also an excellent reason for dying.
>
> ALBERT CAMUS, 1942

Because it's there, you climb a mountain. Each step up in altitude corresponds to a decrease in air pressure. At 18,000 feet the pressure is approximately one-half what it is at sea level, and that means every time you suck in air to fill your lungs, you are getting only half the amount of oxygen you would get with a breath of equal size on the beach in Miami. Your body has to adjust to running with less oxygen, and if it doesn't, you may die of high-altitude illness.

Why You Die

Almost everyone who climbs high experiences some of the discomforts of less oxygen: headache, nausea, fatigue, lassitude, loss of appetite, loss of sleep. Some humans go further and start collecting fluid in their lungs, a condition known as high-altitude pulmonary edema (HAPE). Why the fluid collects is not exactly known, but it is well known that if enough collects, you'll have difficulty breathing, even at rest, along with chest pain and a productive cough. If you don't lose altitude soon enough, you'll drown in water from your own body.

Other humans at high altitude, more typically at extreme heights, collect fluid in the brain, a condition called high-altitude cerebral edema (HACE). A loss of coordination, sudden splitting headache, loss of normal mental acuity, and bizarre personality changes precede the point where your brain is squished to death by the rising pressure inside your head.

To Live

The single most important thing you can do to increase your chances of living at high altitude is ascend no faster than your body can acclimatize to the decreasing air pressure. If you start feeling bad, stop ascending until you feel better. If you don't start feeling better, go down. Humans who descend almost always recover.

> Moral: There's a reason for living
> way down in the valley.

120

ABUSED BY AVALANCHE

The art of living well and the
art of dying well are one.

EPICURUS, THIRD CENTURY BCE

Anytime you have a mass of snow on an inclined surface, you can have an avalanche. Avalanches come in two types: a loose-snow avalanche that releases from one point and fans out as it descends, and a slab avalanche that breaks off along a long fracture line and descends in great tumbling chunks. Snow slides most often on slopes of 30 to 45 degrees, and even though avalanches occur on slopes of every orientation, they rumble off north- and east-facing slopes more often than south- and west-facing slopes. Broad slopes that curve down into "bowls" and narrow slopes confined by terrain collect the most snow and avalanche the most dangerously. Avalanche danger is greatest during and right after a heavy snowfall. A primary indication of avalanche terrain is evidence that an avalanche has occurred there before: rubble at the bottom of a slope, a fracture line at the top of a slope, the absence of trees when nearby slopes are forested, and trees with the uphill branches ripped off.

Why You Die

Avalanches can kill you in two ways: They can bury and suffocate you, or they can slam you around until your neck or skull or some other really important body part breaks.

To Live

If you don't want to die, there are several things you can do, besides stay home: (1) When you feel the snow starting to slide, rush horizontally to a safe spot or at least to a spot where the force of the slide will be less. (2) If you're caught, throw off everything cumbersome and start swimming like mad. (3) Scream once, but after that keep your mouth shut so it doesn't fill with snow. (4) If you're buried, start struggling toward the surface as soon as the sliding snow starts to slow down, or at least try to clear out a little breathing room for yourself in case someone is looking for you.

Moral: Most death-dealing avalanches
are triggered by the human they kill.

121 | CAPPED BY CARBON MONOXIDE

> Death will come anyway,
> whether you are afraid of it or not.
>
> JOHANN VON GOETHE, AROUND 1830

Carbon monoxide (CO) is an invisible, odorless, tasteless, nonirritating gas, and you don't even know you're inhaling it—until you've inhaled a lot. The gas is the result of incomplete combustion of any carbon-based fuel such as gasoline, kerosene, natural gas, charcoal, or wood. Outdoor stoves, for example, burn inefficiently in an enclosed space, such as a tent, where there is inadequate oxygen. And carbon monoxide poisonings account for approximately one-half of the deaths by poison in the United States every year, making CO the leading cause of fatal poisonings.

Why You Die

Once inhaled, CO enters your blood, where it is approximately 200 to 250 times more bondable than oxygen to the hemoglobin of red blood cells. Hemoglobin normally carries oxygen to the cells of your body. With CO attached, hemoglobin can't carry as much oxygen and can't release what is attached as efficiently. As the amount of attached CO increases to as little as 10 percent of the maximum potential, you'll develop a terrible headache, nausea, vomiting, and a loss of manual dexterity. By 30 percent add irritability, impaired judgment, and confusion. You'll find it increasingly difficult to get a full breath, and you'll start to grow drowsy. At 40 to 60 percent, you'll lapse into a coma. Levels above 60 percent are usually fatal, and the cause is usually heart failure.

To Live

When the bad things first start to happen, move to fresh air. You will probably recover completely in a few hours. If you wait too long, though, you might die even in fresh air. You'll need a high flow of supplemental oxygen, and maybe a hyperbaric chamber, to survive.

Moral: In with the good air, out with the bad.

122 DRIED OUT BY DEHYDRATION

Time is a great teacher, but
unfortunately it kills all its pupils.

LOUIS HECTOR BERLIOZ, 1856

Since you are more water than anything else, and since you lose water all day long (see "Hardboiled by Heatstroke"), you have to take in water, usually by drinking it, to stay okay. When you lose more than you take in, you are dehydrating. If you dehydrate too much, you die.

You know you lose internal water when you sweat, pee, and poop. That loss will be increased with diarrhea and/or vomiting. Danger, too, lies in the wild outdoors when you cannot find adequate water from natural sources. Those little blue lines on a topographical map may be dry beds when you get there.

Because early dehydration often goes unnoticed, be aware of increased thirst and a dry mouth. As dehydration grows worse, you usually start to feel weak, maybe lightheaded, and you become confused. Don't be surprised if your head hurts and your heart pounds. You could faint. Things are really bad when you pee little or nothing and you stop sweating.

Why You Die

You have a couple of choices: Your blood, being mostly water, provides a great lot of the water lost when you dehydrate. If your blood volume drops too low, your blood pressure drops too low and you die of shock. Losing internal water means you're also losing electrolytes that you need to keep your organs working properly. When your heart stops functioning properly, it beats erratically and can stop beating altogether.

To Live

Drink enough water to keep urinating often. Drink enough water to keep your urine light yellow or gin clear. But do not drink too much water (see "Hampered by Hyponatremia").

Moral: Eat, drink, and be merry.

123

ENDED BY EARTHQUAKE

Not all the preaching since Adam has
made Death other than Death.

JAMES RUSSELL LOWELL, 1868

Any sudden release of energy in the earth's crust that causes
the ground to shake is called an earthquake. Most of them are
produced when a couple of the plates making up the earth's
surface move against each other, which they are constantly
doing. An estimated one million earthquakes occur every
year. On the low end of the Richter scale (where most earthquakes fall), say, a magnitude of three or less, you may not

notice the quake. Above that magnitude the ground noticeably shakes, and by magnitude seven it is displaced. The more the ground shakes and ruptures, of course, the more damage occurs. Bad stuff happens not only due to the severity of the earthquake but also according to how close you are to the epicenter. But earthquakes can also cause landslides, avalanches (see "Abused by Avalanche"), fires, floods, and tidal waves (see "Tswept Away by Tsunami").

Why You Die

An earthquake creates numerous ways to expire, but discounting related incidents such as fires and floods, you are most likely to die from being significantly crushed by something falling on you.

To Live

Earthquakes cannot be predicted with great accuracy, but you can find out if you're in an earthquake zone. During a quake, if you're inside a building, stay there. Get out of the kitchen and under a sturdy piece of furniture away from windows. Drop, cover, and hold on. In your car, pull over, stop, and stay inside. Outside, move to an open area away from power lines, tall trees, cliffs, or anything that could fall on you—and lie down.

Moral: Trembling is not always
a sign of nervousness.

124

FRACTURED BY A FALL

He that dies pays all debts.
WILLIAM SHAKESPEARE, 1611

According to people who are supposed to know this kind of thing, falling off of something is the world's second leading cause of accidental death. (To qualify for the first leading cause, you have to be in a moving vehicle that very suddenly stops moving.) Some other people who know stuff say falling off of something in the wild outdoors might be the leading cause of accidental death. Important factors related to whether you survive a fall include how far you fall (a great distance works against you), what you land on (rocks are a poor choice), and your orientation when you land (head first not recommended).

All things considered, it might come down to whether your time is up or not. Climbers have crawled away from a fall of 60-plus feet by landing on their feet. Reports thought verifiable tell of people falling outstanding distances of more than 60 feet, landing on their side, and living. On the other foot, hikers have slipped off a wet log, hit their head, and died.

Why You Die
When the numbers are tallied, the greatest chance of death follows the breaking of a faller's spine, the neck being an

especially dangerous part to snap. Also, a large quantity of dead people who were recently falling died because they tore open their aorta and bled to death.

To Live
Don't fall. Don't even put yourself in unprotected places where you can fall.

Moral: It's as easy as falling off a log.

125

FOOLED BY FROZEN WATER

There is only one way to be prepared
for death: to be sated.

HENRY DE MONTHERLANT, 1932

Every year thousands of winter enthusiasts wander out onto frozen lakes and rivers to fish through the ice, to skate or ski, or sometimes, like the proverbial chicken, just to get to the other side. Most of them get away with it, but now and then some are fooled, thinking the ice will support their weight when it won't. Springs beneath the surface and swirling winds over the surface sometimes create thin ice and danger that is often difficult to detect until you plunge through. And lakes buried in snow may be covered with surprisingly thin ice because the snow insulated the surface of the water, preventing it from freezing solid enough to support you. And rivers rushing beneath ice typically fail to freeze solid enough to hold up a human. Before the plunge you may hear warning cracks, but you often suddenly find yourself in water numbingly cold enough to paralyze you.

Why You Die

Many people mistakenly believe hypothermia (see "Hindered by Hypothermia") deprives you of life in minutes in ice water. Not so. It takes at least a half hour for your body core temperature to drop to the point of hypothermia, even in the iciest aquatic environment. What happens is this: The cold makes you suck in a sudden lungful of air, but your head is underwater, so you suck in water and drown. If your head is not underwater, you panic, flail around a few minutes, then sink and drown anyway.

To Live

Don't panic. Use the first minute to calm down and get your breathing under control. Use the next 10 minutes, the average time left for useful movement in ice water, to attempt to swim up onto ice that can still support your weight. Don't stand. Crawl to safety. If you can't swim up onto the ice, at least reach across the ice far enough to freeze in place with your head out of the water. Maybe someone will find you before hypothermia has time to kill you.

Moral: Thick, in many instances,
is better than thin.

126   HARDBOILED BY HEATSTROKE

Death is but an instant, life a long torment.

BERNARD JOSEPH SAURIN, 1768

If your body produces heat faster than it sheds heat (see "Hindered by Hypothermia"), you can cook your brain to death, the final result of a condition called heatstroke. Your internal fluid level works more than anything else to keep you cool, so getting dehydrated ranks as the primary pathway to heatstroke. You can dehydrate (lose internal water) in several ways: sweating, peeing, pooping, and even breathing. If you're used to the heat, you can lose up to one and a half quarts in one hour while doing something strenuous. But you can also exercise so hard that you make heat faster than you get rid of it, especially in hot and humid environments, even when you are adequately hydrated.

Why You Die

For you to be officially heatstroked, your core body temperature has to reach 105 degrees Fahrenheit. Before you reach that temperature, you'll probably feel hot, tired, headachy, and maybe dizzy and nauseated. By the time you hit 105 degrees, your skin will be very red and very warm to the touch. Your skin may also be dry, but in exertional heatstroke your skin is usually still wet with sweat. Your brain will have altered significantly from normal, leaving you bizarrely different from the person you used to be. At 107 degrees or so, your brain cells start to quickly die. After enough of them die, so do you.

To Live

When you're hot and tired, take a break, drink water, find some shade, or take a dip if water lies nearby. With a brain at 105 degrees Fahrenheit, it's usually too late to take care of yourself. Someone needs to cool you off by removing your heat-retaining clothing, pouring on lots of water, fanning you, and massaging you until you cool down. Then you need a doctor since high internal heat often causes other organs to fail.

> **Moral:** No matter how you mean
> it, being cool is important.

127 HAMPERED BY HYPONATREMIA

A thing is not necessarily true
because a man dies for it.
OSCAR WILDE, 1889

Deeply rooted in the brains of many, probably most, out-doorsy types is this message: You have to drink plenty of water. Some of those types, though, have not gotten another critical message: You can drink too much water. You can drink so much that you dilute the sodium level in your body. That's bad because you have to have sodium to keep water levels (inside and outside of cells) and electrolyte levels balanced. You also need it for your muscles and nerves to work correctly. With water intake too high and/or sodium intake too low, you get hyponatremia—which sort of means "low sodium." It can kill you.

When your sodium is low, you feel unusually tired, restless, and grumpy. You'll suffer weakness, and your muscles may start cramping. Don't be surprised by a headache and nausea; you might vomit. Other people could call you confused. All of that stuff will seem relatively mild if you suffer a seizure and slip into a coma.

Why You Die
When your internal water levels are unbalanced, your cells start to swell. This is bad enough in other parts of your body,

but when they start to swell in your brain, the pressure inside your head increases. Too much pressure and the blood flow to your brain cells diminishes, and when the flow diminishes too much, your brain stops working . . . forever.

To Live

Drink water, yes, but be sure to maintain an intake of sodium. You can do it with regular salty snacks, such as trail mix with salted nuts. Mixing water with an energy drink that contains salt, such as Gatorade, will also work. If you think you are hyponatremic, stop drinking fluids. Eat salty snacks and rest until you feel okay.

Moral: Pass the salt.

128 HINDERED BY HYPOTHERMIA

Your teeth chatter from the cold. Faint shadows
that you are, how wrong it was to go to the
trouble of giving you separate names. Your
dying breath barely tarnishes the air . . .

UGO BETTI, 1953

From the food you eat, your body manufactures energy for
living, with heat as a by-product. You produce so much heat
that your blood would boil several times a day if you didn't
naturally and involuntarily shed the heat through cooling
mechanisms: radiation, evaporation, convection, and conduc-
tion (see "Hardboiled by Heatstroke"). If you expose yourself
to the cooling mechanisms, you'll keep on shedding heat even
when you aren't producing very much, and the warmth at the
core of your body (normally about 98.6 degrees Fahrenheit)
will start to drop. Medically, a drop in core body temperature
to 95 degrees Fahrenheit is called hypothermia.

Although medical science describes hypothermia as a core
body temperature of 95 degrees or lower, things happen before
you reach that point. The first thing to happen is a loss of mental acuity: You get stupid. Signs of stupidity include not put-
ting on rain gear when it starts to rain, not eating when you're
hungry, not drinking water even though you know you need a
lot, and not stopping to set up camp even when it gets too dark
to see the trail. You may have trouble with fine-motor activities

like zipping up your parka. At around 95 degrees you'll start to shiver. The shivering will get worse and worse, and you'll have trouble with gross-motor activities like walking, so you'll sit down or lie down and keep losing heat to the environment.

Why You Die

Suddenly the shivering stops because you no longer have enough energy to shiver. You've run out of gas. Your heart rate and breathing rate will slow down and down, and your muscles will begin to grow rigid. You won't care because you're stupid. Some hypothermic humans who have been warmed from being this cold claim they began to feel comfortable, warm, and sleepy as they neared death. Soon you'll lose consciousness. You can live for many hours in this profound hypothermic state, but eventually your heart will stop.

To Live

In conditions that could cause hypothermia, dress appropriately, in clothing that traps body heat while wicking moisture away from your skin. Drink water often to stay hydrated—enough water to keep your urine clear—and eat regularly to keep your internal fires stoked. Pace yourself to prevent fatigue and heavy sweating. And if you feel even a hint of hypothermia, stop, get dry, and get warm.

Moral: Intelligence is only skin deep, but stupid goes clear to the bone.

129

LIT UP BY LIGHTNING

To die with glory, if one has to die at
all, is still, I think, pain for the dier.

EURIPIDES, CIRCA 455 BCE

When warm, moist air rises rapidly to great heights, dark clouds filled with static electricity tend to form. A charge accumulates on the bottom and an opposite charge on the top of the cloud and on the ground beneath the cloud. When the difference between the charges reaches a potential greater than the ability of the air to insulate, lightning stretches out to equalize the difference. As a direct current, the bolt can reach 200 million volts and 300,000 amps, and a temperature of 8,000 degrees Celsius.

Lightning lights the skies over the earth approximately eight million times every day, roughly one hundred times per second, an astounding number of discharges of electricity of which you will see very few. The bolts fly from ground to cloud, from cloud to cloud, within a cloud, and of course from cloud to ground.

Why You Die

Lightning can kill you in five ways. (1) A direct strike can turn you immediately into something akin to a large, over-done potato chip. (2) Lightning can "splash" on you from off of something nearby that is more attractive than you, say a tall tree, and short-circuit your heart and breathing. (3) The ground current from a nearby strike can enter your body, or (4) you can be in contact with a long conductor, such as a fence, when lightning strikes it, and both ground current and long conductor will have the same effect on your cardiopulmonary system as a "splash." (5) You can be blasted by the exploding air of a nearby strike and thrown against an object, say a tree or rock, with enough force to permanently put out your lights.

To Live
Don't be a lightning rod. Avoid being the highest point around: on top of a mountain or open ridge, at the edge of a

large body of water, out in the middle of an open field. In a storm hunker down, arms wrapped around legs, on insulating material in a stand of trees of uniform height (not touching a tree) or in low, rolling hills. If you're in a vehicle, stay there with the windows rolled up.

Moral: Always hike with someone considerably taller than you—but not too close.

130

QUENCHED BY QUICKSAND

There is nothing after death, and
death itself is nothing.
SENECA, FIRST CENTURY CE

Anywhere on earth you find a tract of loose sand that lies low and stays permanently wet, you may be looking at quicksand. It can be at the bottom of shallow water in a pond or lake, or it can be covered with debris such as dry sand or leaves, and in both instances the quicksand is disguised. The sand is too loose to support your weight and too thick and mucky to allow easy extrication of your body once you have partially sunk. Some quicksand is really quick, and some is rather slow. In any case, if the quicksand is deeper than you are tall, you may drown.

Why You Die

After your head goes under, you'll hold your breath as long as you can, then you'll inhale a bunch of sand and lose consciousness, and in a few minutes your brain will shut down totally. If you do not sink in over your head, you'll have to stand around until you die of starvation. Either way, you have saved the cost of a gravesite.

To Live

Once caught in almost any quicksand (except the very quick-est), you can throw yourself flat on your back and float, gently swim to the edge, and crawl out. But all your movements should be slow. Thrashing around wildly substantially increases your rate of sinking.

Moral: Never get in over your head.

131 STAMPED OUT BY STARVATION

There is a remedy for everything;
it is called death.

PORTUGUESE PROVERB

First, the serious stuff: According to the United Nations, approximately 21,000 human beings die of starvation every single day. The great majority of the daily dead are children, and the age group most affected includes kids five and under. The number of people who starve to death in the United States every day, by the way, totals pretty much zero. Some Americans go to bed hungry, yes, but not enough to die. What starving people have in common is this: They are not consuming enough calories to maintain the energy level life requires. If the problem continues, eventually life goes away.

To die of starvation in the outdoors (or indoors) demands a large time commitment. How long? The general guideline of four to six weeks fails to apply in all cases. If you're big and relatively healthy in the beginning, you might hold out for 12 weeks. Some folks have lasted longer.

And you need to be separated from food. Getting lost in a wilderness with no idea what wild foods you can safely consume will probably work, especially if no one searches for you.

Death by Nefarious Nature

Why You Die

Without food consumption, your body begins to eat itself, and there's nothing you can do about it if you can't eat something not you. Your fat goes first. When the fats are depleted, your body eats your protein, so there go your muscles. Your heart, being a muscle, hangs on the longest but finally stops working. In case you're wondering, this process causes pain.

To Live

Eat something other than yourself.

Moral: Food for thought is not enough.

132

SUFFOCATED BY SUBMERSION

> Death is like a fisherman who catches
> fish in his net and leaves them for a
> while in the water . . . the fisherman will
> draw him up—when he thinks fit.
>
> IVAN TURGENEV, 1860

Several factors shed a bit of light on why 9,000 humans or more die from drowning every year in the United States. (1) Many of the dead were nonswimmers. (2) Most of the drowned victims were not wearing personal flotation devices. (3) Some of them were whitewater paddlers not wearing helmets who hit their heads on the way down. Some of them *were* wearing helmets and hit their heads on the way down. (4) At least one study estimates that more than half of the dead had alcohol or some other mind-altering substance "on board." (5) The loss of core body temperature and/or the loss of coordination from being immersed in cold water were factors in a large number of drowning incidents. (6) Males drown far more often than females, with males outnumbering females 12 to 1 in boating-related drowning accidents.

Why You Die

Those who die during a submersion incident typically go through a series of events that vary little from individual to individual. The person panics and struggles fiercely while

Death by Nefarious Nature

holding his or her breath. The heart rate speeds up and the blood pressure rises. Involuntary swallowing of water is common. Swallowed water may or may not cause vomiting. The drive to breathe becomes overpowering, and the person inhales water. Asphyxia, an inadequate intake of oxygen, causes a loss of consciousness. Respiratory arrest and then cardiac arrest soon follow.

To Live

To avoid becoming a statistic, see above and stay calm. If you pull someone from the water and he or she is not breathing, you should start rescue breathing as soon as possible. In the absence of a heartbeat, start CPR.

Moral: There is much value in keeping your head above water.

133

TWISTED BY TORNADO

> The worst evil of all is to leave the
> ranks of the living before one dies.
>
> SENECA, FIRST CENTURY CE

Thunderstorms and hailstorms are related to tornadoes and classified as "locally severe storms." Local storms routinely display high winds, but tornadoes go further, spiraling inward and upward in a vortex that can be of incredible power. The bottom of the vortex (the funnel) can be several yards to several hundred yards wide and reach up from several yards to more than a mile high with the roar of a closely passing jet. The top of the vortex consists primarily of water droplets, and the bottom of dirt and dust and anything else the wind sucks up. Tornadoes occur most often and most devastatingly in the United States and are most likely in spring and summer. Tornadoes have shredded strips of countryside a mile wide and more than 100 miles long. They have picked up loaded freight cars from trains and thrown them through office buildings. They have ripped houses into tiny pieces. They have driven straws through trees. They have taken little girls and dogs from Kansas to Oz.

Why You Die

Your greatest opportunity to die in a tornado comes when you stand outside, exposing yourself to whatever the storm has turned into a speeding missile: boards, bricks, limbs of trees, cows, small imported cars. You can also be picked up and turned into a speeding missile yourself, your demise coming shortly after you are slammed into the ground or anything else standing in your flight path.

To Live

Stay inside a building, away from all windows, in the basement (if there is one) or in a center room. If you're in a vehicle, drive away from the funnel, but don't wait out a tornado in a vehicle. Move inside a building or find shelter in a ditch or low spot. If you're caught in the open, flatten yourself as much as possible against the ground, facedown, with your arms and hands covering your head and neck.

Moral: Adding a new twist to
life can be dangerous.

134

TOPPLED BY TREEFALL

> Death never takes the wise man by
> surprise; he is always ready to go.
>
> JEAN DE LA FONTAINE, NEARLY 1600

Planet Earth can boast of approximately three trillion trees. If that seems like a lot, keep in mind that a mere 10,000 to 12,000 years ago this world had twice that many. Even so, currently there grow woody and leafy just about 400 trees for every human being. And they're not dangerous, right? They just stand there offering shade, and maybe firewood, and sometimes fruit—except several hundred times per year when a big limb or a whole tree falls down on the head of a human, ending that human's life.

Big chunks of wood have fallen "out of the blue," you might say, on campsites, tents, picnic tables, and even on moving objects such as hikers. High winds often, but not always, get the blame. Sometimes someone chopping down a tree cuts wrong, and the tree falls the wrong way, and *wham*—sort of like the revenge of the tree.

Why You Die

A great weight crushes and/or breaks a part of you without which your life is impossible.

To Live

Look up. Do not dally, especially in windy conditions, under "widow makers," dead limbs or dead trees that could possibly land on you if they fall.

> Moral: You will not likely ever see
> a poem as deadly as a tree.

135

TSWEPT AWAY BY TSUNAMI

> Life and death appear more certainly ours
> than whatsoever else; and yet hardly can
> that be called ours, which comes without
> our knowledge, and goes without it.
>
> WALTER SAVAGE LANDOR, LIKELY 1824

The word in Japanese means "harbor wave," and a tsunami is often called a tidal wave, but these mightily destructive rushes of seawater have nothing at all to do with tides. They are the result, most often, of the shifting of geologic faults in the floor of the sea. They can also be caused by huge underwater or land-into-water landslides and underwater volcanic eruptions. Not a single wave, tsunamis are series of waves, sometimes more than 10. Unlike everyday waves, which may reach speeds of 60 miles per hour, tsunamis have been clocked at nearly 500 miles per hour. While normal waves roll along about 300 yards or so apart, the successive crests of tsunamis may be as far as 90 miles apart.

Although a tsunami passing under a ship at sea may go almost unnoticed, the waves slow and increase in height as they near the shore. The first sign of impending danger is typically a sudden rush of water away from shore, leaving a long stretch of seafloor exposed and fish flopping helplessly on the bared bottom. Then the mad rush of water rolls toward land, maybe as a high wall and maybe not. Failing to stop

Death by Nefarious Nature

where the sea usually stops, the tsunami keeps on coming inland. The record tsunami rose 1,740 feet above the high-water mark and rushed 3,600 feet inland, above the average high-tide line, in Lituya Bay, Alaska, in 1958.

Why You Die

You don't have to be outdoors to be killed by a tsunami, but it helps. Waves can get you coming and going. The inland rush of water may be great enough to raze everything in its path and tumble you along until you have drowned. But if it misses on the first try, the wild withdrawal of a tsunami back into the sea irresistibly sucks everything with it.

To Live
Unfortunately, tsunamis often arrive unannounced. If the sea suddenly recedes dramatically, run as fast as you can for high ground or, should one be nearby, the highest floor of a tall building.

> **Moral:** Never camp less than
> 3,600 feet from the ocean.

> Death, the most dreaded of evils, is
> therefore of no concern to us; for while
> we exist death is not present, and when
> death is present we no longer exist.
>
> EPICURUS, THIRD CENTURY BCE

During every moment of every day, about 1 out of every 10 human earthlings is somewhere where a volcano can get him or her. Approximately 600 volcanoes are currently labeled "active." Thousands more are "dormant," which means they could go active any second.

Volcanoes are vents or "chimneys" that lead from the enormous reservoir of molten magma inside the earth to the surface. When gases build up beneath a volcano to the point where something has to give, the molten rock gives because it's softer than the surrounding hard rock. The volcano erupts, and lava flies everywhere. You may think that lava provides your best chance to die, but that isn't true. Lava actually moves so slowly that it is the rare human who can't outrun it. But volcanoes have several ways to make you no longer exist.

Why You Die

You have four ways to go: (1) Falling ash can bury you, a problem that becomes especially likely if it happens to start raining, since rain makes the ash heavy. (2) Pyroclastic flows are horizontally directed blasts from a volcano, blasts that contain ash and hot lava fragments. These horizontal blasts are a flood of fire traveling at great speed, a force that vaporizes everything in its path. (3) Debris (ash and lava fragments) collects near the top of a volcano, and if it gets wet, say from rainfall or snowmelt, it turns into a material similar in consistency to really wet concrete. If the stuff starts to slide, it has been known to travel as far as 60 miles, burying everything in the line of flow. (4) Volcanic gases, which may slip out even when no eruption is taking place, often contain carbon dioxide and other unbreathable stuff, which can settle into low-lying spots and choke you to death.

To Live
Be one of the 9 out of 10 who is somewhere else.

Moral: If you can't take the heat,
get away from the chimney.

137

WITHERED BY WILDFIRE

> A man, when he burns, leaves only a
> handful of ashes. No woman can hold
> him. The wind must blow him away.
>
> TENNESSEE WILLIAMS, 1951

Wildfires—large, sometimes huge, areas involved in uncontrolled flames—have been a part of the natural history of this planet since long before any humans were around to observe them, or even smarter, to move well away from them. From the scientific study of such fires, a relatively recent area of research, experts now divide wildfires into three classes: ground, surface, and crown. Ground fires burn grass and other low-lying vegetation. Surface fires burn grass, low-lying vegetation, and the trunks of trees. Crown fires climb all the way up trees, reaching their crowns (tops), and then rage across the top of the forest. Crown fires are the most destructive—and the most dangerous.

Wildfires burn with the greatest intensity where there is, of course, the most fuel. They also burn uphill speedily and downhill slowly. They are encouraged the most, however, by wind. High wind will turn a little flame into a big flame in an amazingly short time.

Why You Die

Caught in a wildfire? Fear the flames, but the superheated air, which will sear your lungs and/or otherwise make it

Death by Nefarious Nature

impossible to breathe, will kill you before your remains even begin to char.

To Live
Once fully involved, a wildfire typically moves faster than you can run. Sand, gravel, and rocky areas will provide some protection, but your best bet is to find a wet area—swamp or bog—and lie down, seeking a pocket of cooler air to breathe. Or even better, find a lake or river in which you can tread water until the danger passes.

Moral: It's better to burn out than to burn up.

DEATH BY SPITEFUL SPIDER

Wherever you happen to be sitting, or standing or lying, at this moment, a spider almost undoubtedly hides no more than a few feet, and certainly no more than a few yards, away. Spiders dominate the invertebrate predator world and, masters of adaptability, live everywhere from 22,000 feet on Mount Everest to below sea level in the hottest deserts. No fewer than 36,000 species of spiders are known to exist, divided into more than 3,000 genera and 105 families, and—hold on to your DVD of *Arachnophobia*—experts agree at least 36,000 more species of the class Arachnida wait to be described.

138

BEATEN BY BLACK WIDOW

As men, we are all equal in
the presence of death.

PUBLILIUS SYRUS, FIRST CENTURY BCE

Just about all spiders are venomous. They bite with poison that paralyzes and kills their recently living food, which usually was bigger than the spider. But very few spiders have fangs long enough or venom toxic enough to endanger a human. The black widow (*Latrodectus mactans*) is one notable and dangerous exception, the most potentially lethal spider in the United States.

Female black widows—and only the females can kill you—have been identified in all the Lower 48 and Hawaii, but seem more concentrated in the rural South. Look out for a small, shiny, black, eight-legged creature with a bright mark, typically a red hourglass shape, on the underside of the largest body part. Being insect eaters by natural intent, black widows are fond of constructing their webs in insect-abundant places, such as below the holes of outhouses. At one point in history, 88 percent of all black widow bites to humans were reportedly to the dangling testicles of males.

Shy and retiring by nature, these spiders do not attack humans on purpose, but are misled by disturbances to their web or caught off guard by a naked foot stepping on them. Unable to truly bite, they stab and the venom runs down inside their two exquisitely slender, hollow fangs. Although their poison is among the most potent in the world, they carry very little of it, and death to humans is rare.

Why You Die

You will not feel any pain . . . at first. Then an excruciating, charley-horse-type agony will spread from the bite site to your abdomen, lower back, and sometimes down your extremities. You may feel weak, sweat heavily, develop a fever, experience a rapid heart rate, drool, and vomit. After 8 to 12 hours, things should start to ease off. However, if you're having a really bad day, your respiratory muscles will gradually weaken to the point where you can't suck air in . . . and you'll slip painfully to the point of no return.

To Live

Find a doctor. If your life is truly threatened, an antivenin is available. You might also enjoy strong painkillers.

Moral: Look before you poop.

Every fear is fear of death.

WILHELM STEKEL, AROUND ABOUT 1912

A not-so-distant cousin of the black widow, the brown widow (*Latrodectus geometricus*) shares some, but not all, of the family traits. You will, for instance, see the hourglass shape on the underside of the brown widow, but instead of red look for an orange or yellowish color. Smaller in size, the spider can be brown, or tan or gray or mottled, and a black-and-white geometrical pattern adorns the back (and thus the scientific name). An African immigrant and once relegated to Florida, brown widows now scuttle around the Gulf Coast states, Southern California, and probably some other western states. They seem to be spreading, and where browns and blacks run into each other, it's usually the black widow that retreats. Browns share another trait with black widows—powerful neurotoxic venom.

Why You Die

Despite the potency of brown widow venom, a black widow bite (see "Beaten by Black Widow") calls for a much higher degree of concern. Reason: Brown widows inject quite a bit less poison when they bite. The effects of the venom often stay at and near where the spider bit. Human deaths, however, are well documented, and if a brown widow gets blamed for your demise, your final hours will resemble those of someone killed by a black widow.

To Live

Brown widow bite got you down? See a doctor. An antivenin is available.

Moral: Not all kissing cousins should be kissed.

140 FLATTENED BY FUNNEL-WEB SPIDER

> When we are dead, rugs are no
> thicker than a quick-thorn bed.

THEOGNIS, SIXTH CENTURY BCE

One species (*Atrax robustus*) of Australia's funnel-web spiders, a relative of tarantulas, grows large and aggressive, but unlike tarantulas, which have venom that is relatively mild to humans, funnel-web spiders pack a potent punch, enough to drop you in your tracks. The spiders are glossy black on top and velvety black on the bottom. A close look at their bottoms might reveal a few red hairs, but if you're close enough to see them, you're certainly close enough to deserve a bite. Females, larger than males, might grow to as much as 2 inches across. And yep, they build funnel-shaped webs like burrows under logs, rocks, stumps, and dense vegetation. As with all tarantula-type spiders, funnel-web spiders possess fangs that hang down vertically, a characteristic they compensate for by rising up on their hind legs and striking like a snake. The fangs are 4 to 6 millimeters long (about 1/8 inch) and strong enough to penetrate your fingernail or your toenail, making removal of the spider from your body sometimes a problem.

Why You Die

You're going to feel a lot of pain from the bite, due at least as much to the power of the strike as to the venom itself. Within about 20 minutes, however, the pain should spread through your entire body. Another five minutes should produce high blood pressure, rapid heart rate, and increased body temperature. Within two hours you ought to be sweating, drooling, and crying, in company with diarrhea and uncontrollable, weird muscle movements. About this time you'll either start to recover or your lungs and/or heart will stop working.

To Live

Wrap the bitten arm or leg in an elastic bandage and splint the extremity. Stay as calm and still as possible while someone transports you to a hospital where the antivenin awaits.

Moral: You may think it's funnel,
but the joke's on you.

RUINED BY RECLUSE SPIDER

Pain lays not its touch upon a corpse.

AESCHYLUS, NEAR 456 BCE

Brown spiders or brown recluses (*Loxosceles reclusa* and near kin), sometimes called fiddlebacks, are light tan to dark brown in color, grow to an inch or slightly more across, have long legs, and bear a dark violin shape on their top side, with the neck of the violin reaching toward their rear end. They're common in the southern states and up the Mississippi valley and are spreading around the United States. A rather cosmopolitan creature, they are at home in homes: under houses, beneath beds, in the backs of closets, in the sleeves and legs of old clothes you haven't worn for a year or so. But if you're interested in being bitten by one, rest assured they haunt the outdoors as well, preferring to hide out in piles of brush, in old rodent nests, and under logs. Being independent of webs, they hunt at night, stalking their prey. That's when they bite humans.

Stinging pain usually soon follows a recluse bite, but sometimes bitees report no initial pain. Stinging will subside after six to eight hours, to be replaced by an ache and itching that starts around the bite site, which turns red surrounded by white. Fever, chills, weakness, nausea, and vomiting may ruin a day or two. In 24 hours or so a bubble forms, filled with blood or clear fluid. Then a scab forms. Then the scab falls off, leaving a nasty wound that looks sort of like a third-degree burn. It is extremely difficult to get this wound to heal.

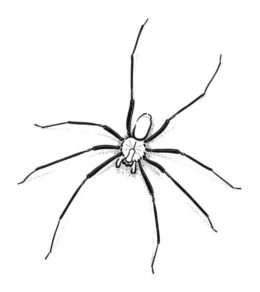

Why You Die

Death could occur in a couple of ways. (1) Infection from the wound could spread throughout your body. (2) The venom could, though only rarely does, disturb the normal functioning of your body enough to cause death. Either way, a fatal recluse bite would put you into a very small category of causes of death. How not boring!

To Live

Recluse spiders do not bite because they think you're food, but because you bump into them with your bare feet, roll over on them while they're crossing your sleeping body, or stick your hand into where they're hiding. If you do get bitten, the care of a physician almost always means you'll live.

Moral: Never fiddle around
with dangerous things.

142 WORKED OVER BY WANDERING SPIDER

> If nothing else, there's comfort in recognizing
> that no matter how much we fail and
> sin, death will limit our suffering.
>
> CHUCK PALAHNIUK, 2014

If asked, and sometimes if not asked, many spider experts will tell you the wandering spiders, also called the Brazilian wandering spiders (genus *Phoneutria*), pack the most dangerous venom of all arachnids. In Greek *phoneutria* means "murderess." Members of this genus can grow to a body length of nearly 2 inches and a frightening leg span of nearly 6. The second from the front pair of legs are hairy, usually, and a dark stripe or stripes runs down the first pair of legs, usually, and a dark stripe runs down the length of the back. You can find them, should that be your thing, in tropical South America, with one species roaming about in Central America. "Wandering" is their name and wandering is their game. They don't maintain webs or hang out in musty lairs. They scurry around the jungle floor at night looking for food: frogs, lizards, and smaller prey. When threatened they become intimidating—rising up tall, raising the front legs, and swaying from side to side. They are not faking.

Why You Die

Bad news: The venom delivered via the fangs of the wandering spider is roughly, oh, twice as dangerous as black widow venom (see "Beaten by Black Widow"). Sort of good news: About two in three bites to humans are dry, venom-less, because the spiders don't want to waste it on large, inedible creatures. If you're in the unlucky one-third, you'll experience severe pain from the neurotoxin they inject. If you're really unlucky, you'll lose muscle control, including the muscles you use to breathe, and you will die of asphyxiation.

To Live

The antivenin is very effective. Find some right away.

Moral: Not all who wander are lost.

DEATH BY FICKLE FATE

Yes, this final section ranks among the somewhat contrived. A scorpion deserves the name arachnid (the eight-legged), but not the title of "spider," so it didn't fit there. And a centipede claims too many "legs" to fit anywhere in this book. Curare, from a poisonous plant, requires injection to do its bad thing, eliminating it from the death-by-edible "vegetable" section. It was either contrive a reason to put these ways to die in other sections or contrive a section.

143 | CENSURED BY CENTIPEDE

Our repugnance to death increases
in proportion to our consciousness
of having lived in vain.

WILLIAM HAZLITT, 1817

Centipedes, those creatures of a hundred feet, differ from millipedes, those of a thousand feet, in a couple of ways. For one thing, centipedes, around 3,000 species, have a pair of feet per body segment (not always exactly 100), while millipedes, about 6,500 species, have two per body segment (which, by the way, numbers a millipede's feet around 200 and a far piece from a thousand). For another thing, centipedes are carnivores and millipedes are vegetarians. Centipedes grab their prey with claw-like jaws and drive in the points of their two modified front legs, injecting venom down ducts in these legs.

Why You Die

When a centipede stings you, it will hurt. If the culprit happens to be a *Scolopendra heros* of the southwestern United States, a centipede achieving 6 to 8 inches in length, the pain can be extreme and the venom can cause serious complications including dizziness, nausea, and collapse, with possible massive swelling near the bite, loss of motor function, and even loss of muscle tissue. Death, so far, appears not to happen with US centipedes.

But in the tropical regions of Asia, centipedes grow to a foot in length and regularly eat small birds and mice for a living. Although information on tropical centipedes is scarce, reports indicate that Indian and Burmese centipedes have kept human victims bedridden for over three months, Sri Lankan centipedes have caused human deaths, and centipedes from Malaysia have stings worse than some of the local death-dealing vipers.

To Live
If it's a US centipede, you will not die, but you might appreciate a strong painkiller. If it's one of those huge tropical centipedes, well, best wishes.

> Moral: Never trust anything with more feet than you and your entire high school biology class combined.

144

CHEATED BY CHOKING

Our last garment is made without pockets.

ITALIAN PROVERB

When you swallow food, it slides down the esophagus (food tube), which when not in use lies flat against the back of your trachea (windpipe). A flap of flesh, the epiglottis, at the base of your tongue covers the trachea when you swallow to encourage food to go down the esophagus. You can, however, get food (freeze-dried pasta primavera should work) stuck in the back of your throat (pharynx), in your voice box (larynx) at the start of your trachea, or even farther down in your trachea. Food that reaches the larynx is often stuck there by a laryngeal spasm, in which the muscles of your larynx constrict to prevent stuff from entering your lungs. Choking can be encouraged by wolfing food only partially chewed, by talking while eating, and especially by having a couple of shots of whiskey before and during dining. Small children sometimes choke on small toys.

Why You Die

Choking can be partial, and you wheeze, moving a little bit of air. Or it can be complete, and you can't breathe, turn blue, often grab your throat, and run away from a group in order to asphyxiate to death in private, cheated out of many good years of life.

To Live

The obstruction can usually be removed by someone who stands behind you, reaches around you, and grasps his or her hands together, placing one hand, thumb in, just above your navel and jerking in and up. This good Samaritan may have to repeat the maneuver a few times to force out the object. You could perform this abdominal thrust on yourself by using, say, the back of a chair or the stump of a tree instead of a rescuer's hands. Internal injuries could result, but at least you'll be alive to heal.

Moral: Chew your food well.

145

CURSED BY CURARE

Our final experience, like our first, is conjectural.
We move between two darknesses.

E. M. FORSTER, 1927

Strychnos toxifera! The name itself should give you an idea of the lethal possibilities of curare, one of deadliest vegetable poisons on earth. Though harmless if swallowed, all of the parts of this climbing vine of Central America and northern South America exude a dark, aromatic, resinous goo that usually brings fatal results if it gets injected into you. The Orinoco Indians inject it into their victims by tipping their arrowheads and darts in the stuff. Theoretically, curare could also cause your death if you rubbed it into an open wound, but it would take a lot. Medical science renders curare into a pure form used in lung surgery, in exacting amounts, to paralyze patients in order to put them on a respirator for the duration of the surgical procedure.

Why You Die

Once inside your body, curare begins its poisonous job of paralysis first on your eyelids and then on the rest of your face. Within seconds you won't be able to swallow or even lift your head. Soon your diaphragm will stop working, and you will find it extremely difficult to breathe. Your pulse will drop like a rock from a cliff. You will turn a ghastly shade of blue, and your dramatic contortions as you attempt to draw breath will soon cease. The series of events surrounding your death occur so quickly that an antidote, even if one existed, would have no time to work.

To Live

If someone was able to keep up your respirations artificially for long enough, it might give your body time to deal with the poison—and you could, at least theoretically, survive.

Moral: Never give offense to the Orinoco.

146

GONE BY GUN

The funny thing about facing
imminent death is that it really snaps
everything else into perspective.

JAMES PATTERSON, 2005

Here's some good news: Your chances of dying from a gun-shot wound in the outdoors are on the decline. Of course, it's only good news if you don't want to die from a gunshot wound in the outdoors. The damage done by the bullet that hits you, whether it deals death or not, depends on several factors, including the size of the bullet, its speed, and where it hits you. Modern bullets often pass right through the victim, puncturing a small hole where they enter and leaving a gaping hole where they leave due to their size and speed. Even smaller bullets can tumble or fragment and blast out a big chunk when they exit the body. In some circumstances you might be the hunted, if you have a tendency to piss off the really wrong people. It is much more likely your death by gun will be an accident.

Why You Die

If the bullet hits something vital—say, your brain or heart—you will be dead right there. It could tear through your lungs and your ability to breathe will slowly or quickly go away. Given the size of your body compared to the size of a vital organ, chances are good you'll be left alive, with big holes out of which you'll bleed until you die.

To Live

When left alive, at least temporarily, you or someone else needs to apply direct pressure to one or both holes until the bleeding stops. Then find a hospital. Oh, and wear bright orange during hunting seasons.

> Moral: Most of the stuff folks worry
> about isn't going to happen.

147

HASSLED BY HELMINTH

Those most like the dead are
those most loath to die.

JEAN DE LA FONTAINE, POSSIBLY 1688

Helminths are wormlike parasites that take up residence inside a human being. They are found around the world, primarily in tropical and subtropical countries, and are estimated to live in the guts of approximately one out of every three human earthlings. Since most species of intestinal worms, and there are many (see "Tricked by Trichinosis"), don't reproduce while inside you, you can provide habitat for several stringy worms for long periods of time and never know it. Obviously, not everyone dies from internal helminth infestations, but thousands do every year, mostly children and mostly in less-developed countries.

You can swallow the eggs of the worms, which subsequently hatch inside you, when you eat meat or vegetables infected by some types of these worms. You can also suck them off your infested fingers if you touched the eggs. You can be bitten by insects that are carrying some of the worms. Some of them can actually "worm" their way through body openings.

Roundworms of numerous species—including tapeworms, whipworms, and hookworms—are the most common parasitic worms worldwide, with residences well established in a staggering one out of every four humans, including millions of Americans, again mostly children, who are infected with the most common roundworm, the pinworm.

Why You Die

It could happen this way. After the eggs hatch in your small intestine, the larvae crawl through the mucosa to enter your bloodstream, eventually ending up in your lungs, where they rupture through into your alveoli and squirm up your trachea, where you swallow them a second time for a return trip to your intestines. Some helminths will live out their lives quite happily in your intestines, with some species reaching a foot or more in length, mating and laying more eggs, which you poop out. They begin to interfere with your normal gut activity, and you get more and more tired. Your stomach starts to ache, and diarrhea sets in. After a while you die from the inability to absorb nutrients.

To Live

Both the freezing and thorough cooking of food kill helminths. If you get infected, certain drugs can effectively kill the worms.

Moral: It pays to not get too eggs-cited.

148

LATCHED ONTO BY LEECH

Why is it that we rejoice at a birth
and grieve at a funeral? It is because
we are not the person involved.

MARK TWAIN, 1894

Evolved from the same source as the earthworm, 650 or so species of leeches offer a variety of colors, shapes, and sizes, all of which are wormlike, swimming, slimy, bloodsucking life forms. Fortunately, only about 10 percent of leech species can bite through human skin. Of those that can, the hugest leech of all is the secretive giant leech (*Haementeria ghilianii*), last studied a few years ago in the marshy land of French Guiana. Greenish-brown gobs of goo, giant leeches grow to 18 inches. One giant leech could feed on you to the point where you got kind of woozy. Two could probably feed until you passed out. Three might kill you. But nobody knows for sure because it's difficult to get volunteers to put up with the pain and blood loss. Should you choose to investigate, your death could be valuable to scientific research.

Why You Die

When you disturb leech-infested water, they'll undulate over, congregate, and explore you with their puckered mouths. Leeches seek out warmth, the source of their favorite food:

mammalian blood. If you pass the meal inspection, they'll attach with a rear sucker and start gnawing through your skin with the front sucker, which contains three serrated jaws formed in sort of a star pattern. They'll suck blood until they've added as much as nine times their starting weight. Little leeches suck out a little blood. Huge leeches suck out a lot. Little leeches don't hurt much and, in fact, you may not know they're feeding. Huge leeches hurt a lot.

Widely known throughout Southeast Asia, a small leech (*Dinobdella ferox*) prefers to crawl up the nasopharyngeal (nose and throat) passage and feed in the back of the throat of mammals, including humans. Theoretically, enough of them could slime in to choke you. Nobody knows about that for sure either.

To Live

Use your fingernail to break the seal where the leech's mouth is attached. Then wash the wound with soap and water. Unlike most bloodsuckers of the world, leeches carry no disease-causing germs transmissible to humans. But the wound stays open longer than most due to an anticoagulant in leech saliva, so watch for signs of wound infection.

Moral: There's a sucker born every minute.

149

NUMBED BY NAEGLERIA

After all, what's a life, anyway?
We're born, we live a little while, we die.

E. B WHITE, 1952

A single-celled living organism, a species within the genus *Naegleria*, this microscopic do-badder lives up to its nickname: the brain-eating amoeba. Loving heat, it multiplies in warm freshwater such as ponds, rivers, and especially hot springs. It can live in warm soil, too. To cause infection, it must go up your nose. Swallowing it is harmless. On the upside, many people expose their noses to this amoeba every year, but infections are rare. On the downside, 97 percent of people infected die.

Why You Die

When *Naegleria fowleri* gets sucked up into your nose, it attaches to nerve tissue and takes the shortest route possible up into your brain. Even when traffic is heavy, it's a quick trip. Although mostly a bacteria-eating amoeba, this one will start to consume your brain. In about two weeks you'll start to show the first signs and symptoms of naegleriasis: headache, fever, nausea, vomiting. Then your brain will start malfunctioning. You'll be confused, unable to pay attention, and you'll wobble because your balance goes. You might have

Death by Fickle Fate

a seizure, and you might hallucinate. At the end of a third week, too much of your brain will be gone for life to continue.

To Live
Never snort the water when you're swimming or soaking in warm, untamed lakes and springs. If you think you have naegleriasis, get to a doctor. A drug with a slim chance of curing you exists.

Moral: The nose knows.

150

STUNG BY SCORPION

Oh Death where is thy sting?
It has none. But life has.

MARK TWAIN, 1894

Nothing much, or perhaps nothing at all, has changed for scorpions in the last 400 million years or so, give or take a few millennia, except there are far more feet trying to stomp them to death. Arachnids (relatives of spiders), they still scuttle rapidly on eight legs, with lobster-like pincers to grab and rend their prey and a five-segmented "tail" which is actually the end of their abdomen. A single sharp stinger at the end of the tummy has two orifices of extremely small size fed by two relatively large venom glands. Scorpions are nocturnal and solitary, often aggressive, and sometimes deadly to humans. Found almost everywhere, scorpions are most common in the tropics and in other warm climates. Of the approximately 650 species of scorpions worldwide, about 40 species are known to scuttle in the United States. Of those 40, only the attractively slim, sculpted, and pale yellowish *Centruroides exilicauda*, found in the Southwest, has been known to end a human life, usually that of a child. Death by scorpion is far more common in India, where species such as the dreaded, dangerous, and darkly black *Palamneus gravimanus* lurk in every other nook and cranny.

Death by Fickle Fate

They will sneak into your tent or sleeping bag and hide in your clothes, in your boots, and under rocks, bark, and leaves. When the abdomen curls up, the scorpion is ready to sting with the speed of greased lightning. The result is almost instant pain from the compelling poison, which attacks the victim's nerves.

Why You Die

As the toxin from a deadly scorpion takes effect, the localized burning pain may spread to your abdomen, and you'll curl up in sheer torture. With cold and clammy skin, you will shiver and shake, sweat profusely, and vomit violently several times. You will have increasing difficulty breathing as you slip closer and closer to respiratory failure. Finally, 12 to

15 agonizing hours later, with frothy fluid bubbling from your nose and mouth, you will slough off this mortal shell.

To Live

If you know you're in scorpion country, look before you put your hands or feet into dark places, and shake out your clothing and boots every morning and your sleeping bag every night. If you get stung, the application of cold usually eases the pain. Antidotes for scorpion venom are being tested, so you might want to wait to get stung.

Moral: A tail may be more than a tale.

ABOUT THE AUTHOR

Buck Tilton, a wilderness medicine expert, cofounded the Wilderness Medicine Institute and has authored many FalconGuides, including *Wilderness First Responder*, which earned an award for excellence from the American Medical Writers Association. He also wrote three books under the Globe Pequot Press's how-to imprint Knack, one of those being *Knack First Aid*. He lives in Lander, Wyoming, and teaches English at Central Wyoming College.